THE**FOOD**DOCTOR
for babies & children

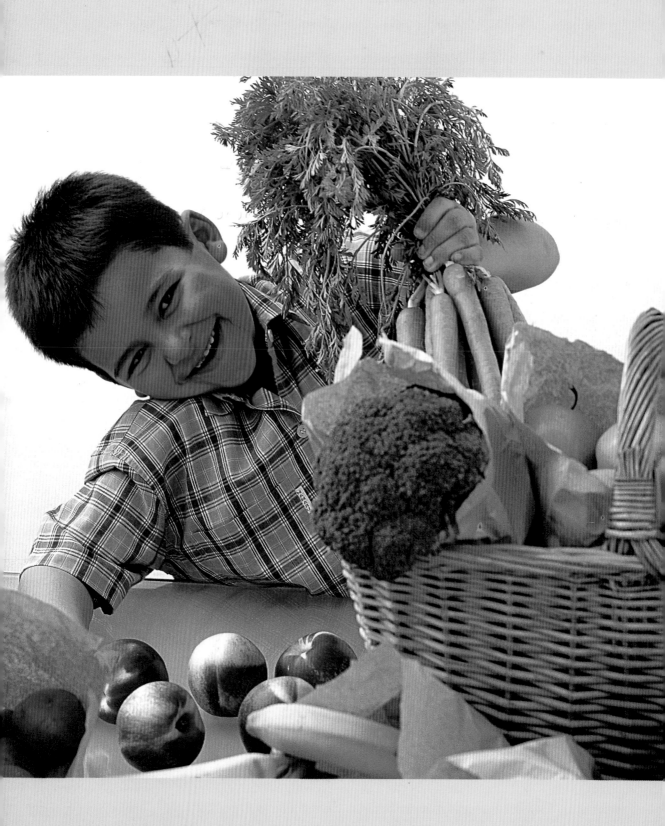

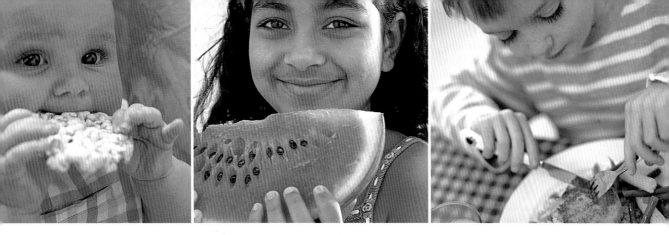

THE FOOD DOCTOR
for babies & children

Nutritious food for healthy development

Vicki Edgson

for more information on nutrition visit

www.thefooddoctor.com

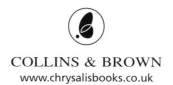

COLLINS & BROWN
www.chrysalisbooks.co.uk

For Flo and Ollie, Jack and Shelley

My sincerest thanks go to Juliet Dennis for her superb research skills, Claire Wedderburn-Maxwell for endless encouragement, and Colin Ziegler for not giving up on the author!

With many thanks to the following models and their mothers: Flo, Ollie and Shelley Greensted, Sam Morgan and Clare Graham, Isabel and Clare King, Mimi and Juliet Dennis, Maya and Varsha Sanderson, Eric, Juam and Ellie Jay, Naadirah Qazi, and Lara Bhogal.

First published in Great Britain in 2003 by
Collins & Brown Limited
Chrysalis Books
The Chrysalis Building
Bramley Road
London W10 6SP

A member of **Chrysalis** Books plc

British Library Cataloguing-in-Publication Data:
A catalogue record for this book is available from the British Library.

ISBN 1 84340 000 6

Managing Editor: Claire Wedderburn-Maxwell
Editor: Mandy Greenfield
Design Manager: Liz Wiffen
Designers: Sue Miller and Liz Brown
Photographers: Daniel Pangbourne and
Nicki Dowey
Home Economists: Sara Lewis and Jo Garside

Reproduction by Classicscan, Singapore
Printed and bound by Canale, Italy

9 8 7 6 5 4 3 2 1

SAFETY NOTE
The information in this book is not intended as a substitute for medical advice. Any person suffering from conditions requiring medical attention, or who has symptoms that concern them, should consult a qualified medical practitioner.

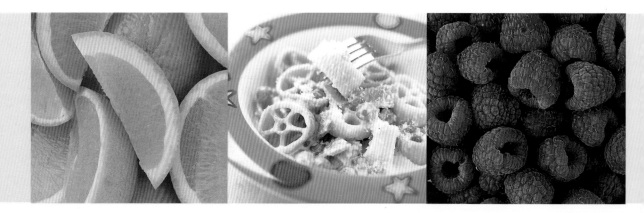

Contents

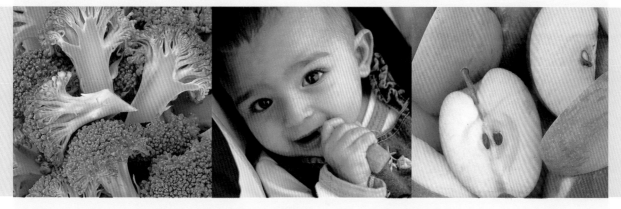

Foreword

by Dr Mike Thomson

I am a paediatric gastroenterology consultant and the father of two – soon to be three – small children. In both of these roles I cannot recommend *The Food Doctor for Babies & Children* highly enough.

This book gives sensible, practical, everyday advice, based upon a sound scientific background for parents in today's confusing nutritional world. It deals with common fallacies and fads very well, exploding nutritional myths where they occur – and, let's face it, there are plenty of misconceptions and myths in children's nutrition in our modern world.

Hopefully it will allow both new and experienced parents alike to get some feel for a healthy diet for their children while not making us, as parents, become too obsessive about the nutritional intake of our children. The mealplanners are particularly useful if, like me, your culinary imagination is exhausted after one or two days. It is important not to become hostage to the guilt trips that many of the influences from would-be helpers, and those well-meaning family and friends, not to mention the media in our society, promote about our children's diets.

The Food Doctor for Babies & Children provides a sensible, practical aid to ensure that your child has a balanced, nutritionally sensible diet, with easy tips on how to administer and prepare for this without being too didactic about nutritional micro-issues. The basis behind nutrition, vitamins and minerals is clearly explained, and on finishing the book I was left feeling that my own children's diet is wanting in some areas. However, this book provided me with the tools to address those issues in a practical and helpful way.

I am sure that all parents and carers alike will find this book to be an extremely valuable resource in the battle to get our children to eat properly and sensibly in today's difficult fast-food world.

Dr Mike Thomson

MB ChB DCH FRCP FRCPCH MD
Consultant in Paediatric Gastroenterology and Nutrition
Centre for Paediatric Gastroenterology
Royal Free Hospital
London, NW3 2QG
www.paediatricgastroenterologist.com

The saying 'we are what we eat' could not be truer than for our children.

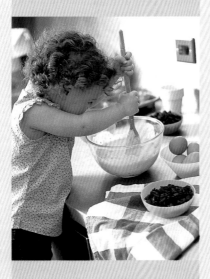

Introduction

The difference between a child who is simply fed daily and one who is optimally nourished is immeasurable. Mental alertness, sound sleep, boundless energy without hyperactivity, and a virtual absence of illness are the norm in children who are receiving the nutrition they need to blossom and flourish.

Inevitably there are many conflicting views, and the theory that 'grandma knows best' often wins the day. However, credence should also be given to the huge amount of research now being carried out into the functional aspects of the bodies and minds of growing children. The saying 'we are what we eat' could not be truer than for our children. The enormous growth of the fast-food market over the last 10–15 years, coupled with the vast increase in the incidence of weight problems, begs the question: is there a link between the quality of our food today and the rise in obesity?

Knowing what a child needs for his or her optimum function and growth is the responsibility of every caring parent, and we at the Food Doctor have aimed in this book to provide you, the parent, with easy-to-access, relevant information that enables you to assess those needs. Remembering that each child is individual, you must take into account specific requirements over and above those of the average child, and we would recommend that you seek the help of a nutritional consultant, dietician or doctor whenever special advice is required.

However, in the day-to-day management of your child's feeding and nourishment, we hope we have addressed the fundamentals of nutrition for the formative years. There is no disputing the comparative ease – and negative aspects – of modern-day convenience food, but a better understanding of how you can contribute to a healthier, happier child is our pledge to you in this book.

Ultimately there is no substitute for fresh food, although the mere suggestion sends some people reeling in despair. 'Where is the time to prepare fresh food?' they ask, to which we always reply, 'It only takes as much time to wash an apple as it does to open a packet of crisps.' Fresh food looks good, smells good and always tastes better. The hidden incentive is that it also provides many more nutrients than its pre-packed alternative. However, not all packaged food is bad for your child, and in *The Food Doctor for Babies & Children* we help you sift the good from the bad, so that you can make more informed choices.

We believe that every child should have this chance at the beginning of his or her life, and we wish you, and your child, information, exploration, fun and reward as you browse through this book.

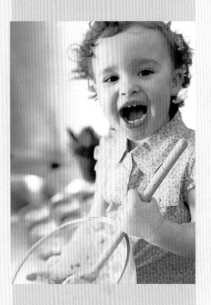

Children who are given the opportunity to help in the kitchen tend to be less fussy in their eating habits.

PART 1

Good food for kids

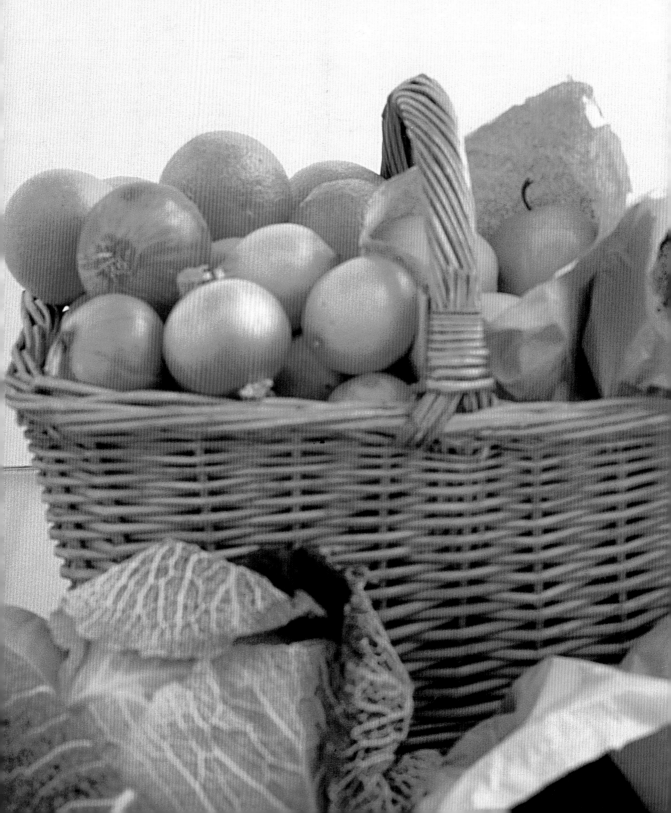

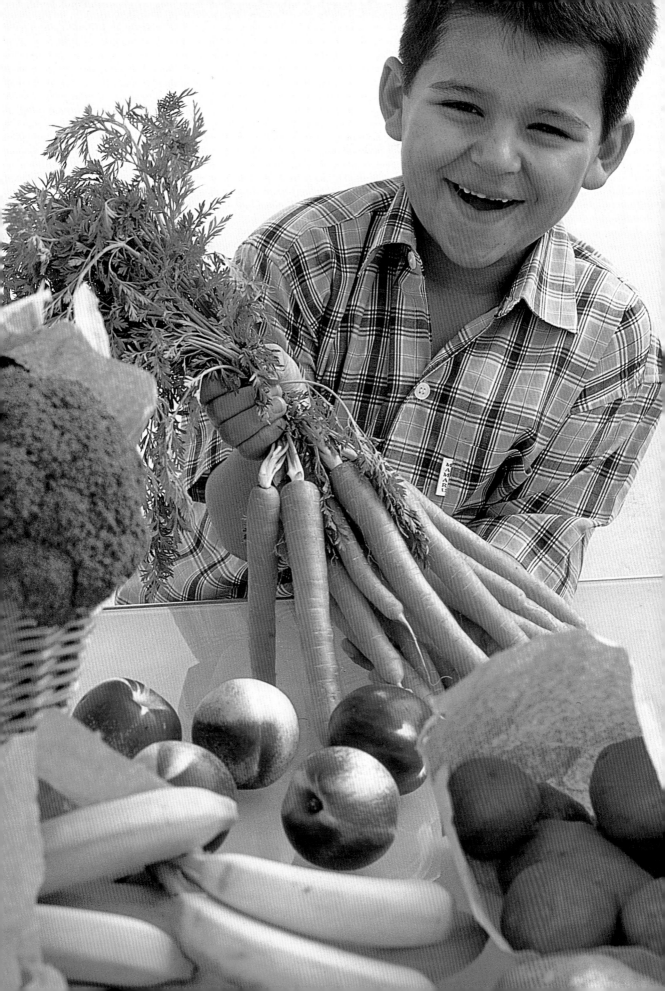

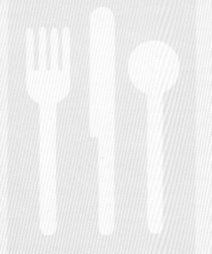

Good nutrition

'Nature cures, when given the opportunity.'

Dr Bernard Jensen, 1988

Good nutrition is the regular supply of a wide variety of nutrients to meet the demands of the body from moment to moment in its development and survival throughout life.

Understanding what is required to build a strong, healthy body demands a few basics in anatomy and physiology. If this sounds complicated, don't despair – we are talking about *basics*, not the minutiae of every cell and its function. We all require a good range of specific types of food to provide us with the building blocks for the multitude of different functions in the body: we need certain foods for our brains, certain foods for our muscles, and others for our hearts and lungs. In children this is particularly important, since from the minute they are conceived and throughout their rapid development they demand all the foods essential for growth.

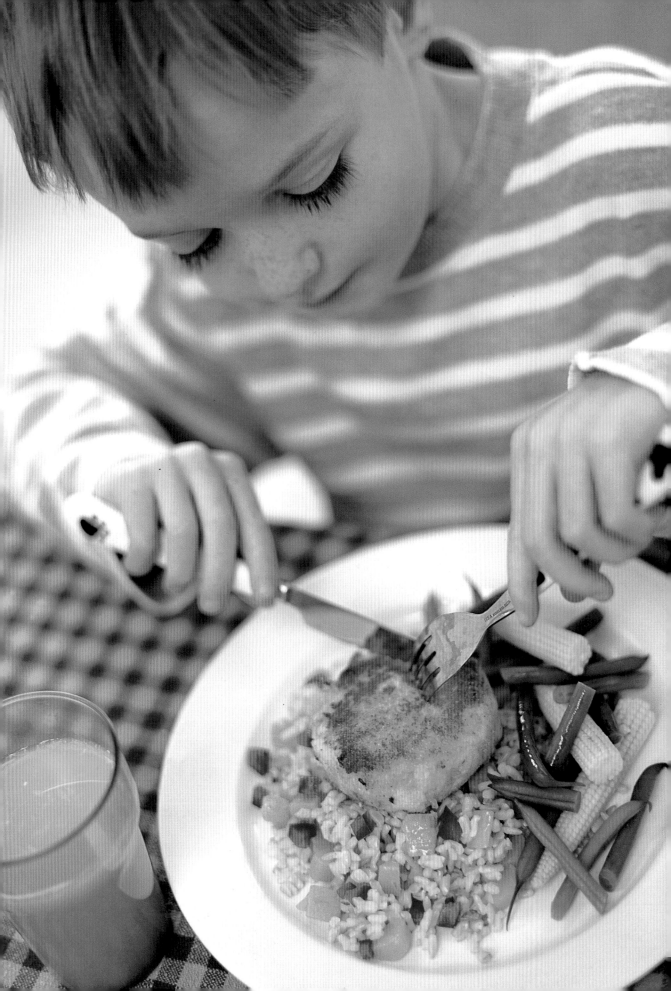

From breast to bottle

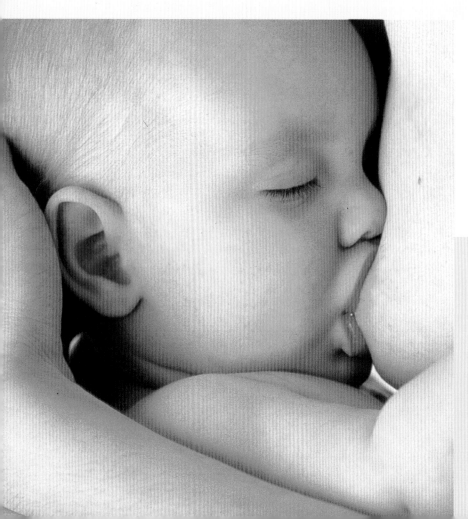

Mothers' breast milk contains all the nutrients a baby needs for development and growth in the first four to six months, as well as specific antibodies that are required in building the immune system, particularly in the digestive and respiratory tracts. A baby is obviously most vulnerable during the first six months of life, and providing breast milk may offer the best protection against potential infections and allergens. Recent research has also shown that breastfed babies have a higher IQ than those given infant formula preparations from birth. However, in some cases it is not possible for a mother to provide breast milk; if breast-feeding is not an option, then professional help will be given to ensure that your baby obtains from a formula preparation exactly what he or she needs.

Reasons for weaning your baby early

- Baby needs more than just breast milk
- Returning to work
- Insufficient milk supply
- Chronic mastitis
- Insatiable infant hunger
- Post-natal depression

Breaking from breast to bottle

In today's busy lives there is a tendency to breastfeed for a shorter length of time than in the past, without considering the long-term implications for the health of your child. The first six months are naturally the most important time, and it is generally recommended that you breastfeed for at least four months to enable the immune system to develop as much as possible, prior to introducing formula milk of any type. Breast milk is so complete that it provides your baby with all the necessary nutrients for complete growth and development. However, other pressures also play a part, especially if you have a large baby who requires more than you are able to provide; in this case it is important to recognize the signs that you need to supplement breast milk with formulas.

It is generally recommended that you wean from breast to bottle over a period of several weeks, to enable the infant's digestive and immune systems to adapt to the changes in nutrient content of the formula milk of your choosing.

> Breast milk is so complete that it provides your baby with all the nutrients for complete growth and development.

What is formula milk?

Infant formulas have traditionally been based on cow's milk extract, and yet cow's milk bears little similarity to human breast milk. Soya-milk formulas suit some babies, but not all, as soya milk is one of the top ten allergens (substances that promote an allergic reaction) for babies and children. The development, over the last few years, of goat's milk formula has been a vast improvement for those babies who will not tolerate cow's milk formula. Interestingly, it is the higher content of essential fats in goat's milk that is important, preventing cradle cap and eczema in sensitive babies. Goat's milk is actually the closest of all animal milks to human breast milk, and it is for this reason that we recommend it so highly. While these are the best-known formula milks, there are a number of non-dairy casein-free formulas such as Neocate and Pregistimil.

When to wean symptoms

- Your baby is still hungry after feeding
- He is waking in the middle of the night
- Your baby is interested in your food
- She is becoming restless and irritable
- Your baby is listless and excessively tired

Adverse formula reactions

Some formula milks may not be suitable for your baby. Any of the following reactions could indicate an intolerance, in which case it is recommended that the formula is changed immediately to prevent further disturbance.

- Skin rash
- Colic, or pulling the legs up to the chest
- Persistent crying
- Spots on the bottom
- Dry skin, eczema or itchy patches
- Disturbed sleep
- Vomiting
- Swollen lips or mouth
- Wheezing or difficulty in breathing
- Loose, frequent stools

At birth, 14 per cent of a baby's total body weight is fat, rising to 25 per cent by the time he or she is six months old. Providing the correct ratio of fats, including essential fats, is vital for the total health of the immune, hormonal and nervous systems, all of which are fat-dependent.

Formula varieties range from powder preparations, which must be mixed with sterilized water to a specific recipe, right through to ready-formulated milk that can be served straight from the container. Much research is being undertaken to improve the quality and presentation of formula milks, so it is worth searching through your supermarket and local health-food shop to check out all the options. It is essential to follow the manufacturers' instructions on the packaging to ensure the correct nutritional balance for your baby.

If your baby is under four months, it may be possible to top up breast milk with formula preparations to provide sufficient quantity of milk without wearing you out. There are many formula milks on the market today, but the most important thing to recognize is when they are not suitable for your baby. See Adverse formula reactions (page 13) for guidelines indicating a possible intolerance to a formula preparation.

Choosing between different formulas

Casein and whey are both proteins that are found in milk, and it is whey-dominant preparations (approximately 60: 40 whey: casein) that are most similar to breast milk. Whey protein is easier for small babies to digest, and these formulas are suitable for babies under three months. Casein-dominant formulas (approximately 25: 75 whey: casein) are more similar to cow's milk. They are more suitable for larger, hungry babies, because casein takes longer to digest, and will usually provide more satisfaction for the infant.

A question of immunity

As mentioned above, the essential fats found in both breast milk and, to a lesser degree, formula preparations are vital for the development of the body's immune system. Mother's milk provides all these essential fats in the correct proportions for her baby, which vary from child to child. If your baby is prone to frequent colds, infections and allergic reactions, this may be an indication that her immune system is not up to scratch. In some instances, supplementing her diet with a small amount of essential fats from a vegetable source (such as sunflower, linseed or safflower oil extract) may be appropriate, but this should never be attempted without the advice of a nutritionist, dietician or other health-care specialist.

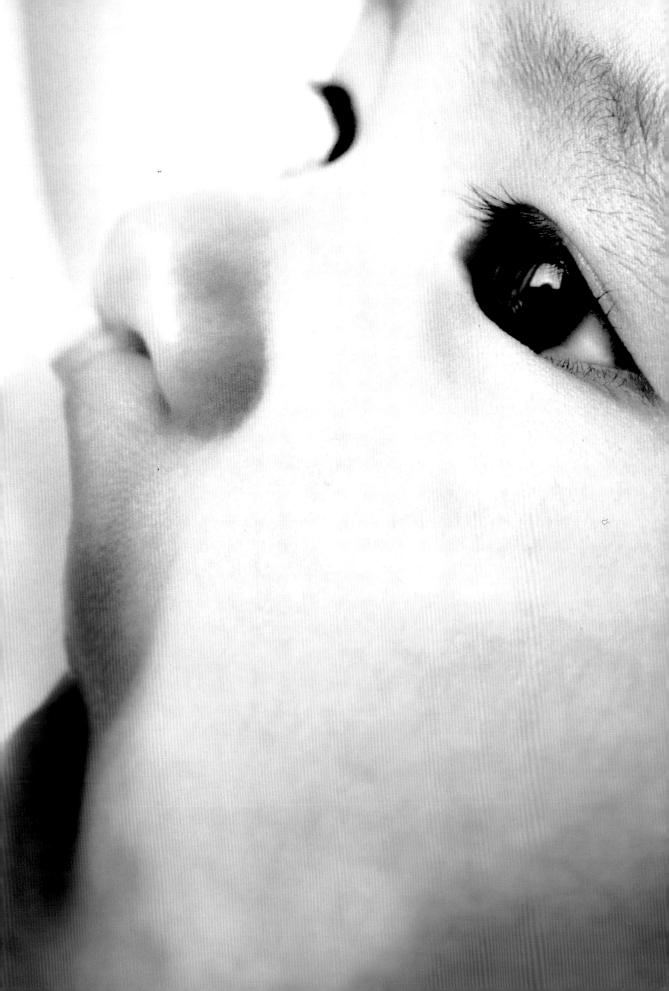

Essential building blocks

Understanding what food is made up of and how it is used in the development of your child is an essential first step in providing optimum nutrition. We have all heard of proteins, carbohydrates, fats and fibre, but exactly how and why they are required in the body is not so well understood.

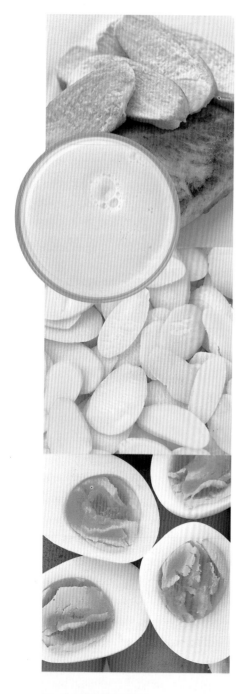

PROTEINS: the body's bricks and mortar

Proteins are vital for the development of the skeletal structure (including the bones, cartilage, ligaments, teeth and nails of your child), as well as for the body's hormonal system and for the chemical messengers of the brain and nervous system.

All animals – whether they fly, crawl or swim – are made up of primary proteins. Secondary proteins are derived from vegetable sources such as nuts and seeds, grains and beans. They are broken down in the digestive tract into amino acids, which are the building blocks of every cell, organ and system in the body. We cannot rebuild our bodies without protein, and in the early stages of development and growth, large amounts of protein are required on a daily basis to meet the demands of the rapidly growing body. The saying 'From small acorns, big trees grow' illustrates the power of protein in building strong, healthy bodies.

The big eight

There is a total of 22 different amino acids, which are the breakdown products from the proteins that we eat. Eight of these are called 'essential', because we cannot make them in our bodies and must therefore derive them from our diet. All animal products provide these eight essentials, but in vegetarian diets it is necessary to eat a combination of nuts, seeds and grains in order to obtain them, as these foods are only 'partially complete' proteins.

Breast milk provides only 1.5 per cent protein, but this is all it takes for a baby to nearly double in size in the first six months. We often mistakenly think that abundant protein is essential, and yet the danger

Best proteins for children

Milk, cheese, eggs, yoghurt, meat, fish, chicken, pulses, lentils, quinoa, millet and oat grains, nuts (except peanuts) and seeds, soya produce (including soya milk and tofu), with smaller amounts of protein derived from vegetables.

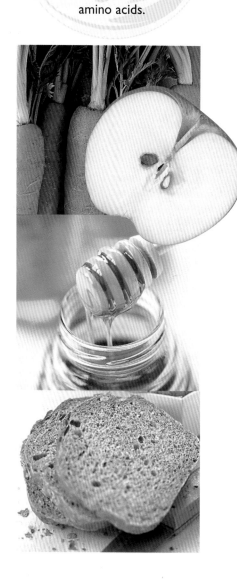

Toddler's top tip

All children need several portions of protein every day, one of which should be from an animal source, to ensure the full quota of amino acids.

at this age is too much rather than too little. Protein produces an acid by-product, and an excess of it can overburden the kidneys of a young child. See the chart on page 81 for weaning and first foods for guidelines on quantities of milk formula you should give your baby.

CARBOHYDRATES: fuel for the body

The body uses carbohydrates for the production of energy and for keeping warm. They are broken down into glucose, which is carried to the muscles, brain and other organs, to enable thinking, movement, speech, breathing and yet more food digestion to take place. Carbohydrates should collectively form the lion's share (approximately 60 per cent) of the daily food intake of any child, and it is important to provide a good range of them in the form of cereals, breads, pulses, rice and other grains, plus a wide variety of fruits and vegetables.

Simple and complex

All carbohydrates are broken down into two main groups: simple and complex. Simple carbohydrates have been processed and refined in order to prepare other products, such as a loaf of bread or a cake made from wheat, rye or other grains. In this processing, however, many of the essential nutrients are lost, and much of the fibre is removed, making the carbohydrates far easier to digest and absorb, but also raising the body's blood-glucose level more rapidly. These are known as 'short-energy' foods as they provide their energy quickly, but it is not long-lasting. See Sugar and spice (pages 38–41) for a more detailed explanation of how this works.

Complex carbohydrates are those grains, pulses, vegetables and fruits that have not been altered or processed, leaving their nutritional content intact. They should form the larger part of a child's daily carbohydrate content, as they are slower to digest and provide energy over a more sustained period.

Carbohydrates: simple and complex

Simple: Bread, pasta, cakes, biscuits, croissants, crackers, pastry, sweets, chocolate bars, crisps, other manufactured snacks, processed breakfast cereals, white rice, sugar, jams, marmalades, jellies, soft drinks.

Complex: All fruits, vegetables, wholemeal flour, wholemeal pasta, wholemeal bread, brown and wild rice, wholegrain crackers and biscuits, wholegrain breakfast cereals, oat or millet porridge, muesli, mixed cereal grains, buckwheat pancakes and pulses.

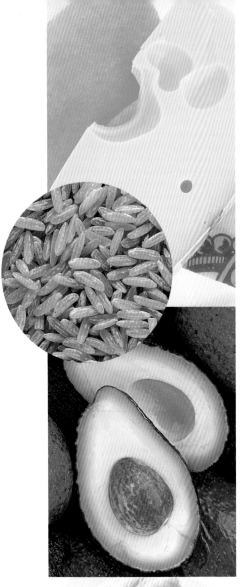

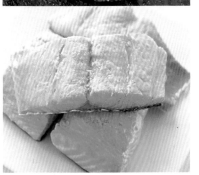

FATS: messengers, carriers and oils for the body and brain

We read so many adverse comments about the fats in our daily diet, without understanding the difference between good and bad fats. It is true that excessive quantities of animal fat and refined sugars (found in sweets, cakes and biscuits) can lead to obesity, diabetes and heart disease in later life, but eating the beneficial fats is essential for good health.

In children, these essential fats are required for the development of the brain and nervous system, the hormonal system and digestive tract, and for the growth of the eye retina. They are needed for a healthy heart and cardiovascular system, and for well-functioning lungs and the respiratory system.

Baby-soft skin

Not all babies have beautifully soft skin, and this is one of the easiest ways to detect an insufficiency of essential fats in the diet. Fats act as a lubricant on the skin, both internally and externally, and if your child is suffering from any kind of skin complaint, it could well be that he is not obtaining or absorbing the beneficial fats from his diet.

Essential fats are so called because they must be derived from the diet and cannot be manufactured by the body on its own. They fall into two main groups, generically known as omega-3 and omega-6 essential fatty acids.

The fatty fats

The fats found in red meat, chicken and other poultry, dairy products and cheeses are all known as saturated fats, rather than essential fats. They also play an important role in the developmental stages, but care should be taken not to overload the infant's digestion with an excess of these fats from too early an age. Too much saturated fat

Essential fats

Omega-3: Salmon, tuna, sardines, mackerel, linseeds, sunflower seeds, pumpkin seeds, sesame seeds, walnuts, wholegrains and chicken.

Omega-6: Almonds, filberts, pine nuts, sunflower seeds, pumpkin seeds, sesame seeds, corn and avocados.

- Some of these fats need to be introduced after the first 12 months to minimize the possibility of allergies. See Part 2 for the stages of development and the recommended introduction of different foods.

will compete for absorption with the essential fatty acids and will inhibit their important functions. It is recommended that one main meal a day includes animal protein (thereby carrying with it the saturated fats), and that the remaining protein is derived from non-animal sources. However, it is important to note that children do require more fats of the essential and saturated forms during the winter months to provide them with the added warmth they need.

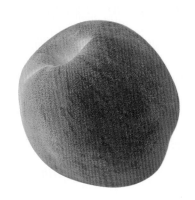

It is now known that a child's fat cells are laid down during the first five years of life, and any child who is overweight for her height at this age is likely to battle with a weight problem for the rest of her life.

FIBRE: the missing link

A healthy diet for children is gauged by efficient digestion, absorption and elimination. A lack of fibre and fluids in the diet constitutes the two main causes of constipation, and of poor elimination through the bowel, kidneys and bladder, as well as the skin. Fibre is found in two main forms in the infant diet – soluble, and insoluble – and both are required for efficient elimination.

Less well known, perhaps, is the function that fibre plays in the role of balancing blood-glucose levels – a major factor in energy production, concentration and the functions of the brain. Fibre slows down the digestion and absorption of carbohydrates, and as such ensures a more even release of energy over a longer period of time. This is explained in greater detail under the Glycaemic index of foods and drinks (pages 38–9).

Soluble fibre is found in fruits and vegetables, and in some grains. But juicing fruit removes its important fibre content, and juice should really only be served with a piece of fruit at the same time. For young infants, fruits and vegetables are puréed to eliminate any lumps that cannot be broken down, without removing the fibre content.

Insoluble fibre is found in the husks of grains such as wheat and rye, which act as a broom to the intestinal tract. This can be abrasive on an infant's underdeveloped digestive tract, and we do not recommend introducing too much grain (other than rice) before 12 months.

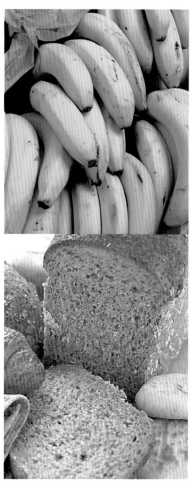

The Food Pyramid

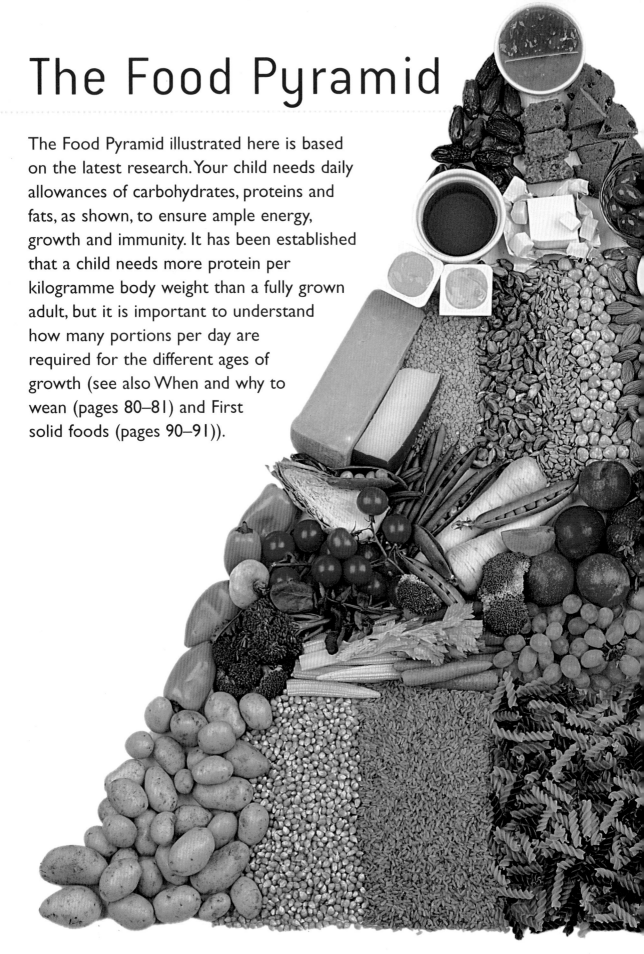

The Food Pyramid illustrated here is based on the latest research. Your child needs daily allowances of carbohydrates, proteins and fats, as shown, to ensure ample energy, growth and immunity. It has been established that a child needs more protein per kilogramme body weight than a fully grown adult, but it is important to understand how many portions per day are required for the different ages of growth (see also When and why to wean (pages 80–81) and First solid foods (pages 90–91)).

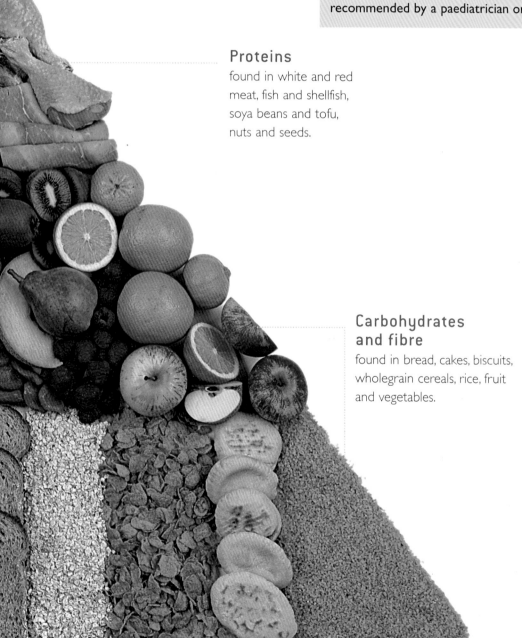

Fats

found in oily fish, red
meat, poultry, dairy
foods, nuts and seeds.

Cholesterol

The recommendation for the total amount
of cholesterol to be consumed per day for
children over the age of five is the same as
for adults, i.e. not exceeding 300 mg per day.
However, before the age of two, the cholesterol levels found in breast milk and formula
milk are important for the development of the
hormonal and nervous systems, so it is vital
that children should not be put on fat-
restricted diets of any kind, unless specifically
recommended by a paediatrician or doctor.

Proteins

found in white and red
meat, fish and shellfish,
soya beans and tofu,
nuts and seeds.

Carbohydrates
and fibre

found in bread, cakes, biscuits,
wholegrain cereals, rice, fruit
and vegetables.

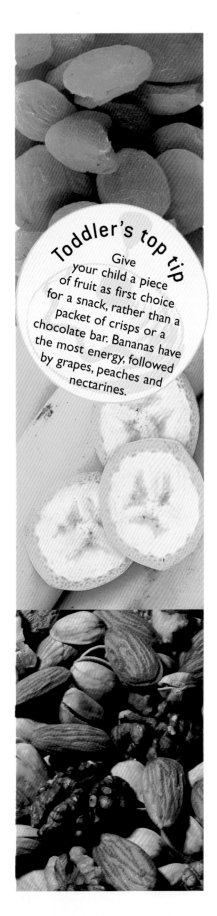

Give your child a piece of fruit as first choice for a snack, rather than a packet of crisps or a chocolate bar. Bananas have the most energy, followed by grapes, peaches and nectarines.

Toddler's top tip

The Food Pyramid

The Food Pyramid will give you a better understanding of what proportions of protein, carbohydrate and fat your child should be eating. It is important to understand which foods fall into which group, and when they might belong to more than one. For example, fish is a primary protein (because it is an animal), but it also falls into the fats category, as it contains essential fatty acids in its oils that are vital for the development of brain tissue, nerves and hormones.

Of sugars – good and bad

You will notice that natural sugars (shown mainly in the fruits section) will meet any child's sugar requirements. It is the inclusion of fast foods and drinks that will tip the scales out of balance and initiate cravings in your child's eating habits that need never have begun.

Dried fruits (such as dates, raisins and apricots) may be used to stave off such cravings, or as foods that provide quick-release energy. However, they should not be given if your child has a tendency towards hyperactive behaviour, because compounds in these fruits have been found to induce over-activity of certain parts of the brain in susceptible children (see Recognizing hyperactivity, pages 70–71, for more on this subject).

Sweeteners (such as honey, molasses and rice or corn syrup) are all preferable to granulated and brown sugars, as the glucose in these highly refined sugars is easily broken down by the digestive system, causing dramatic fluctuations in blood-glucose levels in your child.

Proteins – brain, body and bone builders

All animal foods are primary proteins, and are considered the most important proteins for healthy growth. Fish, chicken, turkey and eggs, milk, butter and cheese (as well as a limited amount of red meat) fall into this category, as does breast milk.

Equally available – although not considered individually to be 'complete' protein – is the wide range of legumes and pulses, such as butter beans, kidney beans, garbanzo beans, lentils and split peas. Such proteins are all inexpensive but highly nutritious sources of essential amino acids (see page 16), which may be added to soups, casseroles, purées and dips, especially where fussy eating is a problem with your child.

Nuts and seeds are also important sources of protein, although care must be taken to ensure that there is no possibility of allergy in the family (see Allergies and intolerances, pages 64–9). Nut butters are a tasty and filling snack food, as well as an excellent accompaniment in lunch boxes.

Essential fats – nurturing intelligence

It is a well-known fact that the body requires energy for brain function, digestion and maintaining the correct body temperature – functions that are even more important in young children than in adults. A hungry child will always be cold and shivering, no matter what the external temperature; equally, loss of concentration can often be blamed on a lack of nutrients to the brain.

Regular meals are vital for young children, and it is important that each meal contains some fats, which are essential for brain function, body insulation and a healthy hormonal system. No child should ever have to be put on a fat-restricted diet unless he or she has been allowed to eat highly sugared foods for several years and has become unnecessarily obese (see Overweight or underweight, pages 52–3).

Beneficial fats are found in fish and lean meat, as well as nuts, seeds and their oils. Including ground pumpkin, linseed and sunflower seeds in your child's porridge or breakfast cereal (mixed in with their milk) will go a long way towards ensuring that they get their daily allowance of essential fatty acids (see First cereals, pages 134–6).

Carbohydrates – the grain of life

Carbohydrates that are grain-based are broken down into complex and simple varieties. These form the largest part of any child's diet, being the most abundant and the greatest source of energy on a daily basis. They therefore comprise the base of the Food Pyramid, and a nutritious diet should be reliant on more of the complex carbohydrates than the simple variety, as these provide more – and better quality – energy.

Complex grains are those that have had minimal processing prior to being packaged. They are rich in nutritional value, providing energy throughout the day and reducing the likelihood of the mood swings and irritability that are often associated with highly sugared foods. They include muesli, porridge oats, wholemeal and wholegrain breads and muffins, cornbread, brown rice, buckwheat noodles, barley and millet.

Simple carbohydrates are those that have had most of their fibre removed and have been bleached, blanched and refined, to provide many of the tempting bread and biscuit-based products that are so readily available today. The main problem with such foods is that, in the processing, most of the goodness has been removed, rendering them almost nutritionally empty. They include most commercial cereals, biscuits, white bread and flour, bagels, pasta, white rice, egg noodles and most pastries. Children are often drawn to these foods because they tend to contain added sugars and colourings, and are often associated with popular television characters in order to increase sales. As well as being addictive, such carbohydrates fill your child up with hollow calories, allowing little room for any of the other important foods, such as fruits and vegetables.

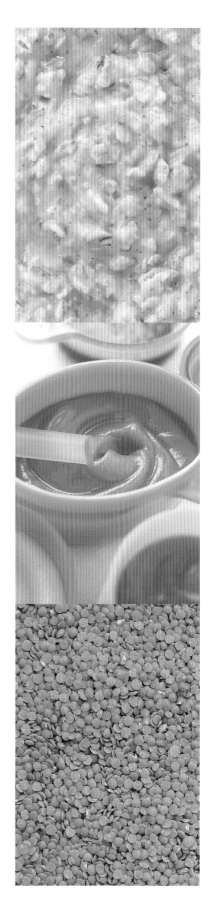

Healthy growth

Knowing what your child needs for the different stages of growth takes you a long way towards a better understanding of his food choices. As most parents know, a child goes through many phases of likes and dislikes in the first few years of life – a source of constant frustration for any dedicated mother!

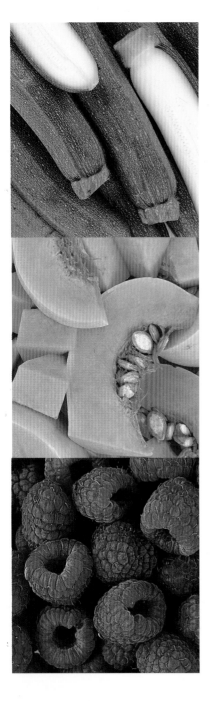

Changes in taste

When a child changes his food preferences seemingly overnight, it is usually an indication that a specific area of growth and development is taking place that may differ in nutritional needs from another area. The best approach is to provide a wide variety of foods throughout all stages, as far as possible. But remember that children are actually far more immediate than adults in their nutritional needs, as around a third of their food is being used for growth and development in the first few years of life.

The breath of life

The complicated structure of the lungs develops throughout the foetal period and the first three years of life. If babies are born prematurely, their lung capacity may not be sufficient to supply their oxygen requirements, and it is not uncommon for premature babies to be assisted in breathing during the first few weeks of life. Full-term pregnancy needs to be reached to ensure optimum lung capacity at birth.

Oxygen is carried in the red blood cells in the circulatory system, from the lungs to the brain and other organs of the body. Iron is the most important mineral for the formation and health of red blood cells, so it is important to ensure a good intake of this mineral on a regular basis during a child's developing years. Children who appear to be mildly anaemic are often also lethargic and lacking in physical energy, and a shortage of iron may explain this (see page 57 for recommendations on the richest food sources of iron). Vitamin C is also required for the uptake of iron into the cells, as well as for the delicate cell membranes, particularly in the tissues of the lungs. As the body cannot store vitamin C, it is important to consume a variety of foods on a daily basis to provide this vital nutrient. As well as citrus fruit, kiwi fruit and watermelon have abundant vitamin C, as do all berries and potatoes, tomatoes, squash and sweet potatoes.

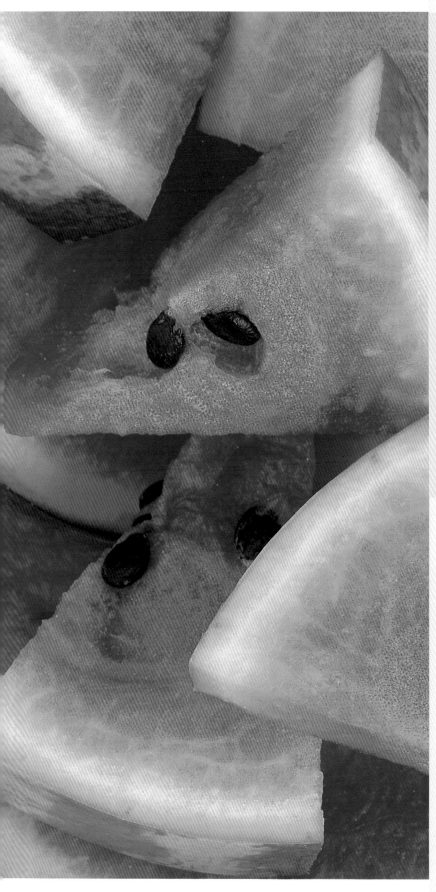

Bone-building

The formation of bone commences from the fourth month in the womb, whereas the spinal column and cranium (part of the skull that encloses the brain) begin their development within the first month. At birth, the spinal column has two main curves, and by puberty this number has increased to four, to support the weight of the head and the remaining structure of the body. (At birth, the ratio of the head to the rest of the body is 1 : 4, while in an adult that ratio comes down to 1 : 8.) This explains why young children often have a deep arch in the base of their spine, with a protruding bottom, which tends to straighten out as they approach their teenage years.

Calcium is the most important mineral for bone-building, and approximately 400mg is recommended daily for optimal growth and for development of spinal and skeletal tissue, as well as teeth. However, magnesium, manganese, boron and vitamin D are also needed in order for calcium to be efficiently absorbed – all of which can be supplied through human breast milk, if breastfeeding is an option. Alternatively, formula milks take these requirements into consideration.

Top 40 foods

The following fruits and vegetables will provide a full balance of nutrients, but please note that the list is by no means exclusive and your child needs a wide variety of foods.

Senses
Immune system
Digestion
Bones
Nervous system
Heart
Hormones
Urinary system

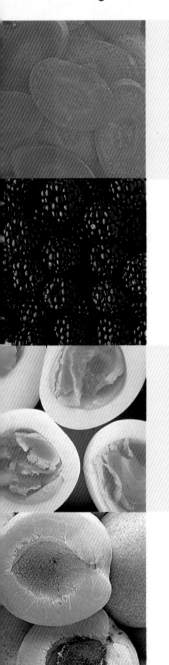

CARROTS

are an excellent source of beta-carotene, which is vital for the health of the inner and outer skin, including the lungs and respiratory system. Beta-carotene converts in the body into vitamin A, which is important for immunity and protection against viruses and infections. Carrots are also rich in potassium and fibre, to ensure proper digestion and elimination. One of the first foods to feed to a baby, as they are naturally sweet.

BLACKBERRIES

These small fruits are a very good source of vitamin C, which is necessary for building a strong immune system and for the formation of collagen, a vital protein constituent of the skin. Additionally, blackberries are rich in beta-carotene for ensuring good eyesight. They may be puréed from fresh or tinned fruit as the nutrient content is preserved in the canning process.

EGGS

are one of the richest sources of vitamin A, for immunity and for skin and eye care. They are also a good source of the B group of vitamins, which are required for energy production and good digestion. Egg yolks contain abundant iron (necessary for carrying oxygen to the brain), as well as zinc (for the immune system) and vitamin D (essential for building strong bones). Providing there are no symptoms of intolerance, eggs are one of the most important foods for young children, and can be included in the diet from nine months old.

APRICOTS

The deep orange colour of these fruits indicates their rich supply of beta-carotene, which is needed for a healthy immune system, good eyesight and healthy skin. They are also one of the richest sources for children of iron, which is necessary for energy and brain fuel. Additionally they have laxative properties, which are safe to use, and their natural sweetness makes them an ideal component for early purées and puddings. Soaking them overnight plumps them up and increases their natural enzyme content. If buying dried apricots, do not choose the sulphured varieties, as these tend to irritate those children who may be prone to asthma or allergies.

AVOCADOS

Actually a fruit, rather than a vegetable, the avocado is one of the richest sources of vitamin E, which is required for immunity, wound-healing and ensuring soft skin. Avocados are also a great source of folic acid, which is needed for the formation of red blood cells in children to prevent anaemia, as well as of abundant B vitamins for energy. They may be puréed or mashed with other vegetables and fruits, and are excellent for weaning and for first food purées and mash.

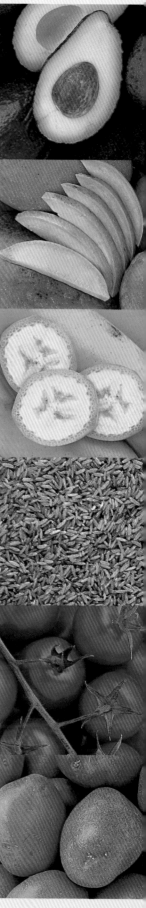

MANGOES

The mango is one of the richest sources of beta-carotene and vitamin C, both essential nutrients for boosting immunity and maintaining healthy skin, hair and eyes. It is also a good fruit source of calcium and magnesium for building strong bones and teeth. Mangoes may also have a calming effect on the digestive system, as they are highly alkaline and help to balance any acidity or upset-tummy problems. They are good for purées and puddings.

BANANAS

One of the most energy-packed foods for children – not just because of their sweetness, but also because they are a rich source of carbohydrates and B vitamins, which are required for the production of energy. Bananas are also a good source of potassium, ensuring a healthy heart, as well as being calming for the digestion by stimulating the growth of beneficial bacteria in the digestive tract. Rice and bananas together are known to be one of the best tummy-settling combinations for children.

RICE

Long known for its benefits as a first weaning food, rice is the staple diet of more than one-third of the world's population. Brown rice is packed with energy-giving B vitamins, as well as zinc for immunity and growth. It contains both calcium and magnesium, which are needed for healthy bones and teeth. It is also an excellent food to relieve tummy upsets and diarrhoea, and the water in which it is cooked is used in the Far East to settle colic in infants. Rice milk is now commercially available in cartons and is a good alternative to those who are allergic to cow's milk.

TOMATOES

are indispensable in the family kitchen, not only for their versatility, but for their highly beneficial nutrient content. Strictly a fruit, not a vegetable, as they are rich in an antioxidant called lycopene, and packed with vitamin C, they are greatly immune-enhancing, However, it should be noted that eating very large amounts of tomatoes can interfere with calcium absorption. As most ketchups (although branded as 'healthy') are very high in sugars, puréed fresh, tinned or carton tomatoes are preferable as a main source.

POTATOES

This hardy root vegetable is packed with energy-providing carbohydrates and abundant B vitamins, as well as being a good source of vitamin C for protecting the immune system. Many children crave potatoes, perhaps for their B3 content, which is required for the 'happy factor' neurotransmitter in the brain, known as serotonin. Keep fried potatoes and chips to a minimum, to avoid destroying the rich supply of nutrients, and opt for baked, mashed and boiled potatoes instead.

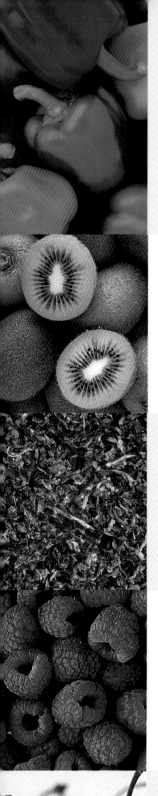

SWEET PEPPERS

Three colours of peppers (red, orange and yellow) contain abundant vitamin C and beta-carotene, which together provide the immune system with essential nutrients. In fact, red peppers have more vitamin C than an equivalent-sized orange, as well as high levels of selenium to add to their immunity value. The green variety is also rich in vitamin C, but does not contain as much beta-carotene. Peppers are also rich in folic acid, to prevent anaemia, and fibre to ensure good digestion and elimination. These vegetables are all excellent as puréed for young infants and in stews and casseroles for older children to add sweetness and fibre.

KIWI FRUIT

These favourites with children actually contain more vitamin C than their equivalent weight in oranges, but may cause intolerance reactions. Their little black seeds provide omega-6 essential fatty acids, which help to prevent skin problems such as eczema. They have inherent digestive enzymes, making them a good fruit for those with sensitive tummies. Soft and sweet, they are one of the best first foods for purées, and can be added to yoghurts for older children or frozen into popsicles.

SPINACH

Long known for its iron content, spinach is also rich in calcium and magnesium, both minerals that are vital for building strong bones and teeth, as well as in potassium, which is heart-protective. Recently it has been found to be a rich source of lutein, a nutrient that improves and protects eyesight, so it should be added to the 'carrots improve your night sight' list. Its slightly bitter taste can be lessened by adding it to mashed potatoes, which also makes for a more interesting mash or purée (see page 131).

RASPBERRIES

Rich in vitamins C and B3, these delicate little fruits are a favourite with children and have a high supply of calcium, for improving bone and teeth strength. They also have natural antibiotic properties and help to alleviate diarrhoea, as well as reducing mucus and phlegm during colds and flu. Raspberries are also known to have anti-spasmodic properties that are helpful in the relief of pre-menstrual cramps in adolescence. They are ideal as part of purées for infants and for natural ice-lollies (see page 147).

CHERRIES

Children find these sweet fruits irresistible and, being rich in vitamin C, they are important for the immune system. Interestingly they have anti-spasmodic properties, and are therefore useful when children have eaten too much of another kind of fruit, producing tummy cramps. They are also one of the richest sources of iron, for preventing anaemia and increasing the transport of nutrients to the brain. They may be eaten fresh, or from a tin – but take care to choose the unsweetened varieties, as they contain enough fruit sugars to preserve themselves naturally.

PEARS

As one of the staple fruits in the family kitchen, pears offer a rich source of vitamin C, to enhance immunity, and folic acid and iron, to protect against anaemia. They also contain pectin, which helps to improve elimination, carrying toxins from the body. They serve as an excellent natural laxative, and are considered one of the best first foods for infant purées, as they have a very low intolerance level. They are one of the few fruits that contain a high level of iodine, which is required by the thyroid gland to enhance metabolism and energy production.

ORANGES

Always known to be rich in vitamin C, oranges also have potent anti-viral and antibiotic properties, making them one of the most popular fruits. Eaten whole, their fibre helps to regulate elimination, preventing constipation. However, oranges are only beneficial when eaten fresh – many of those found in supermarkets are several weeks old, or were picked before they ripened. And freshly squeezed orange juice provided in cartons is often very high in fruit sugars, and can become quite addictive to some children. It is best to offer a range of orange-based fruits, such as satsumas, clementines and oranges themselves, when they are in season, rather than year-round, to ensure that your child does not develop an intolerance.

WATERMELON

Considered by some nutritionists to be the very best source of vitamin C, this Caribbean fruit is also rich in beta-carotene, making it one of the best immune-boosting fruits in the family kitchen. It is also a rich source of potassium, which has heart-regulating properties, and is beneficial for the nervous system. As such, it is ideal for making juices, popsicles and fruit punches for the summer. However, as watermelon is digested rapidly it should be eaten separately from other foods to prevent the possibility of the melon's natural sugars fermenting in the stomach with the other foods.

SQUASH

As with all orange-coloured vegetables, squash are rich in beta-carotene and vitamin C, which are vital for the immune system. Squash are also a good source of iron, which is important for energy and for carrying nutrients to the brain. Both calcium and magnesium (needed for healthy bones and teeth) are found in these vegetables, making them excellent all-rounders in the family kitchen. Infants can benefit from their rich nutrients in purées and mashes, while older children love them as vegetable chips, or baked in the oven, where they become toffee-like and sweet.

SWEET POTATOES

Similar in nutrient content to the squash family, sweet potatoes additionally contain the nutrients of potatoes – that is, vitamin D for bone health and vitamin E for extra immunity and skin health. They are a particularly good source of vitamin B3, or niacin, which is required for a balanced mood, and they make an excellent alternative to regular potatoes for teenage children who are conscious of their weight, but still need energy-providing foods. They make a good first purée food for infants, as they tend to be quite sweet and have a high water content.

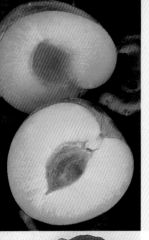

PLUMS AND PRUNES

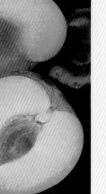 A rich source of iron for children, plums are available in several colours, the darker ones containing a higher level of vitamin C and beta-carotene, for immune-system strengthening. When eaten with their skins, these fruits provide a good source of fibre, encouraging proper elimination. However, an excess may cause diarrhoea, as they do have mild laxative properties. Prunes are dried plums, which tend to have an even higher level of iron, making them an excellent fruit for children who are recovering from illness or weakened in any way. As they are sweet, they are useful for early purées, but care should be taken over the amount that is introduced at the beginning.

TUNA

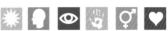 Tuna, an oily fish, is a good source of Vitamin D and calcium. It has an abundant supply of omega-3 essential fatty acids, for hormonal balance, brain function and the prevention of inflammatory conditions such as eczema, asthma and hay fever. As a good source of both vitamin E and selenium, to protect those essential fats, it also supplies the immune system with vital nutrients. In addition, tuna is rich in both vitamins B12 and B3, which are required for the health of the heart and arteries, and for balanced mental function and alertness. Tinned as well as fresh tuna may be used, as all tinned tuna is now taken from fresh fish. Choose tuna that is tinned with olive or sunflower oil for maximum protection.

CAULIFLOWER

 Being one of the brassica family of vegetables, cauliflower benefits from the same nutrients as broccoli, but to a lesser extent, owing to its paler colour. It is also rich in folic acid, which is required for the formation of red blood cells, to ensure a strong cardiovascular system and the carriage of oxygen and nutrients to the brain. It provides a gentle source of fibre for the digestive tract, alleviating constipation, but is high in phosphorus, which can create excessive wind if eaten in large quantities. Introduce it from about five months onwards in infant purées, and use it for bakes and mixed vegetable casseroles and curries for older children.

CHEESE

 As a primary protein, cheese from all sources provides good levels of calcium and vitamin D, for the development of healthy bones and teeth. It is of particular value to vegetarian children who are not eating meat or fish, as it provides some zinc, which is vital for growth and immunity, as well as for good digestion. Only pasteurized cheeses should be given to young children and, as a rule, no cheese should be introduced before six months of age to minimize the possibility of intolerance. A variety of cow's, goat's and sheep's cheese is recommended.

CHICKEN

 As one of the most frequently eaten white meats, and one of the first animal proteins to be introduced, chicken is a primary protein, containing all eight essential amino acids. It is a rich source of vitamins A, B3 and B6 for mental balance, cognitive function and learning; as such, it is an important fuel for the growing body and brain. Chicken is a good source of zinc, for increasing immunity, which is why it is often used in soups. However, care should be taken to buy quality produce, as many of the commercially farmed chickens are now packed with growth hormones and antibiotics – for this reason, it is important to consider buying it in an organically reared state whenever possible.

APPLES

The all-time favourite in any family kitchen, apples provide excellent amounts of vitamin C and beta-carotene, for ensuring immunity, as well as a compound known as pectin, which stimulates beneficial bacteria in the digestive system and removes toxins from the body. If eaten with their skins on, apples provide a good source of soluble fibre to encourage good elimination and prevent constipation in children. Care should be taken in providing apple juice as a substitute for the whole fruit, as in removing the fibre, the juice becomes both excessively sweet and acidic and may cause stomach cramps in some children.

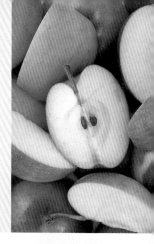

SALMON

As an oily fish, salmon is a good source of calcium and vitamin D, both of which are required to build healthy bones and teeth. Omega-3 essential fatty acids are also inherently found in oily fish, and are vital for hormone development and balance, as well as for the function of the brain and nervous system. The vitamin E in salmon protects these essential fats, and, together with selenium, is important for immune function and healthy skin. Those children with skin complaints such as eczema and psoriasis, or other inflammatory conditions, are often found to be deficient in the omega-3 essential fats, so the regular inclusion of oily fish in the diet is recommended.

MILK

All milk contains large quantities of calcium and vitamin D, both of which are needed to build healthy bones and teeth, as well as playing a part in heart health and growth. However, an increasing number of children are developing varying levels of intolerance to cow's milk, so try either goat's or sheep's milk products instead, as both are now widely available in supermarkets. In rare cases some children are born without the ability to produce the enzyme lactase, which digests the sugar content of milk, making dairy foods a group to be omitted for them. However, there are plenty of other foods, such as eggs, oily fish and dark green leafy vegetables, that may be substituted to ensure an adequate intake of these vital nutrients.

BROCCOLI

One of the richest sources of calcium (one serving of raw broccoli contains more calcium than a pint of milk!) and of magnesium, broccoli is also a source of vitamin K, ensuring strong bone development in children, particularly those who may be intolerant of dairy produce. It is also an excellent source of the B vitamins, as well as of vitamin C, making it one of the true superfoods. It has natural antibiotic and anti-viral properties, as well as providing abundant fibre for encouraging regular elimination. As a green vegetable, it may be introduced early in infant feeding in purées and mashes, and served regularly – either steamed or baked – for older children.

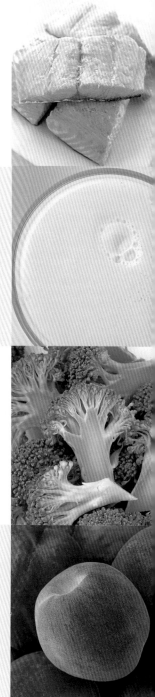

PEACHES

As an orange-coloured fruit, peaches are rich in beta-carotene and vitamin C, both essential for supporting a healthy immune system and warding off viruses and infections. In addition, they are a good source of folic acid, which is required for the production of red blood cells to carry nutrients to the brain and muscles, and for nerve function. When eaten with their skin on, they ensure a good level of soluble fibre to encourage regular elimination, and act as a gentle laxative. They may be prepared in a variety of ways for all ages. As a very alkaline fruit and easily absorbed, they are particularly suitable, when ripe, for children with a sensitive digestion.

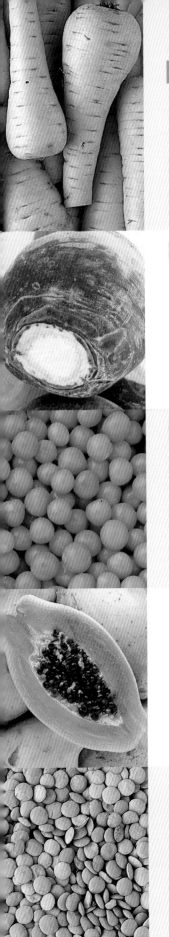

PARSNIPS

These nutrient-rich root vegetables are a great favourite with young children as they tend to be sweet. They have a high potassium content, which is important for the nervous system, and are good for the health of the kidneys and bladder as they have a slight diuretic action. Additionally, parsnips are a good vegetable source of iron, which is needed for energy and to prevent anaemia. They also provide valuable fibre for the digestive tract and help to promote regular elimination. They are excellent in purées and mashes for infants and young children, and roasted for older children.

SWEDES

This root vegetable is actually part of the brassica family (which includes broccoli, cabbage and Brussels sprouts), all of which contain potent antioxidants to protect against illness and infections, including specific compounds that boost immunity against cancer cells. Swede is also a rich source of folic acid and potassium, for the health of the heart and arteries, as well as the nervous system. As the taste of swede on its own is unattractive to some children, it is recommended to mix purées and mashes of it with sweeter fruits and vegetables, such as apple and carrot.

PEAS

Possibly one of the easiest green foods to entice children to eat, these little balls are packed with goodness, including a surprising amount (in a vegetable) of protein, which is essential for the growth of all tissues and organs. Peas are also high in vitamins A and C (for immune function), together with zinc (for growth and rapid wound-healing), as well as magnesium and calcium (for heart health). They are considered a perfect food in their own right, and children cannot eat too many peas. Frozen peas are a valid option, providing they are used within their recommended freezer time. Peas make an excellent first food purée together with carrots or parsnips (see page 131).

PAPAYA

This richly coloured orange fruit is one of the most abundant sources of beta-carotene, which is vital for the immune system as well as for protecting eyesight. But papaya is exceptional in its provision of a natural digestive enzyme called papain, which helps to break down proteins, as well as reducing mucus production and helping to clear runny noses. It also has a strong anti-parasitic action, particularly if the black seeds are puréed with the fruit rather than being discarded, thereby protecting children from thread- and pin-worms. An all-round favourite with children, papaya may be used in purées, juices and puddings (see page 130).

LENTILS

As well as being one of the oldest legumes known to humans, lentils are one of the best sources of vegetable-based protein, containing as much protein as most meats. They also have a very high level of iron, as well as calcium, potassium and magnesium (vital for blood supply and heart health) and zinc (for growth and immunity). They are also rich in B vitamins, for energy production and mental health. Care should be taken when introducing these legumes into the infant diet, as they may be difficult to digest and should not be introduced before 12 months. However, they are an excellent source of protein for vegetarian burgers, casseroles and meat-free bolognese sauces.

SWEETCORN

Traditionally eaten as a major source of carbohydrate in the autumn months, corn-on-the-cob provides an excellent source of B vitamins, which are needed for energy production. The husks of the individual corn kernels provide abundant insoluble fibre (for good digestion and elimination), potassium (for regulating heart health and the nervous system) and phosphorus (for the brain and nervous system). Sweetcorn is rich in magnesium, which is required for relaxing muscles. It is one of the best vegetarian sources of iron, which is needed to prevent anaemia. Rinse tinned sweetcorn thoroughly to wash off excess salt and sugars. Yellow cornflour, or polenta, makes an excellent alternative to mashed potatoes.

OATS

One of the best grains for bone development, containing abundant calcium, magnesium and manganese, oats provide excellent insoluble fibre for aiding digestion and elimination and for clearing toxins from the body. They are also one of the best sources of silicon, which is required for the growth of hair, nails and skin, and which is often lacking in children with eczema and other skin complaints. Also a rich source of B vitamins for energy, and of iron for blood and heart health, oats are one of the most important all-round and versatile foods in a child's diet. Oats can be used in a variety of ways, from cereals to crunchy bars and fruit toppings (see page 145).

RAISINS

Dark raisins and sultanas are simply dried grapes, and as such have a condensed nutrient quality. They are a particularly rich source of iron and potassium, both of which are needed for heart health and protection against anaemia. In addition, they contain abundant magnesium in their skins and are a wonderful natural laxative for children with constipation. Their potassium content is excellent for the kidneys and bladder, and they protect against all infections, as they are rich in vitamin C. Watch out for grape juices in cartons, however, as they tend to be unnecessarily sweetened. Small amounts of natural grape pulp may be included in purées and early weaning foods for added flavour, but take care to remove the seeds.

STRAWBERRIES

These perfect little fruits are irresistible to many children, being sweet, soft and easily absorbed. They are a rich source of beta-carotene and vitamin C (for immunity), as well as folic acid and potassium (for the health of the heart and cardiovascular system, and for the nervous system). Strawberries are one of the only fruits to contain vitamin K, which is essential for calcium absorption and bone strength, thus making them one of the most important berries nutritionally. However, they may be irritating for those with eczema and other skin inflammation tendencies, and care should be taken when first introducing them into the diet, as the tiny seeds on the outside of the berry can be upsetting to undeveloped digestive systems.

  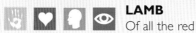

LAMB

Of all the red meats, lamb is often the favourite with children and, as a primary protein, is rich in vitamins and minerals. It is particularly high in iron, calcium and zinc, all of which are required for heart health and the development of strong bones and body structure. The B vitamins are all found in red meat, and lamb is especially high in B6, which is essential for cognitive function and brain health. Being one of the meats that has the least likelihood of causing an intolerant reaction, lamb is often the first red meat to be introduced into the infant diet; it is generally recommended that organic varieties are chosen, in order to avoid the antibiotics and hormones that are often found in non-organic meat.

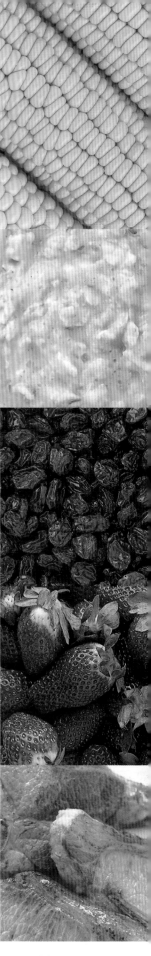

Food choices: good versus bad

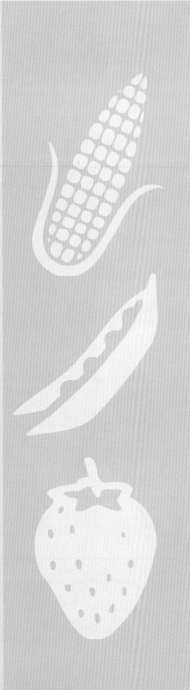

To understand good nutrition, you must be aware of the 'anti-nutrients' – those foods that rob the body of essential nutrients. These are primarily the S and C words: Sugars and Sweets, Salt, Caffeine (as in Colas), artificial Colourants and Chocolates. They appear in almost every type of fun or fast food in one form or another and rob the body of the wide array of vital nutrients found in natural foods.

A well-prepared storage cupboard can be a life-saver, not only on rainy days, but also when other demands prevent you from reaching the supermarket before the little one's hunger pangs set in, such as in the middle of the night during a growth spurt! It is not always feasible, or necessary, to prepare everything from scratch, as long as you have a good under-standing of what will suffice when, and you provide adequate nutritional nourishment.

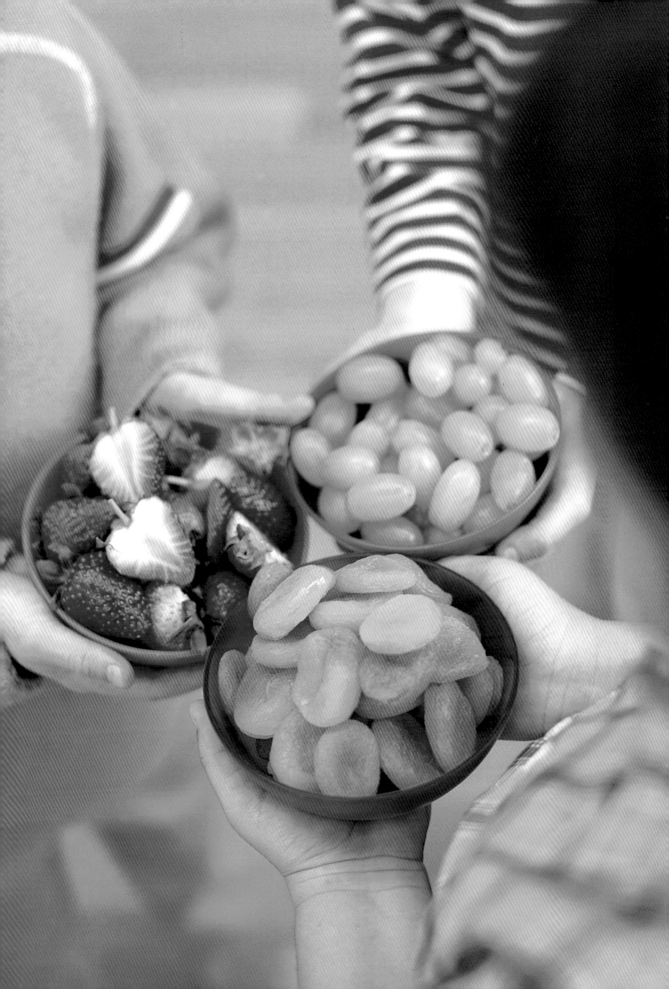

Organic versus inorganic: the debate

The organic baby-food market has grown dramatically over the last five years, with sales in excess of £55 million in the year 2001. In the most recently published Mintel research it is estimated that as much as 40 per cent of the total baby-food market is now organic, compared to 23 per cent just one year ago.

Organic food

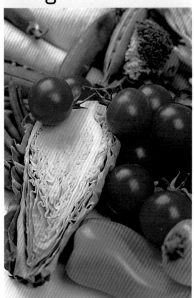

Pros	Cons
No chemicals	More costly
Tastier	Less attractive (fresh)
More nutritious	Less variety

Organic food is defined by the absence of chemical fertilizers and pesticides in growing the individual foodstuffs that make up a product. There are currently approximately 3,000 known chemicals used in our food chain. In the case of fruit and vegetables, there is often a marked difference in the taste of organic food, but the down side is that these fresh foods will not last as long, are often bruised and irregular in shape, and may be less visually appealing than their 'inorganic' competitors.

However, the benefits of introducing such foods as first nutrition for your child are immeasurable because, when weaning, the infant digestive and immune systems are highly vulnerable to new challenges, and an abundance of chemicals may overload them. This can create a greater likelihood of experiencing intolerances and adverse reactions in susceptible children than if organic, unadulterated products are offered as 'first foods'.

During the first year of a child's life the nervous system grows at a very rapid rate, and carries on developing until approximately 18 years of age. Inorganic produce carries toxins that are potentially harmful to the nervous system. The digestion of a one-year-old is actually more efficient and penetrable than that of an adult, making him more vulnerable to the absorption of damaging toxins. Pound for pound, infants consume a much higher percentage of fruits, vegetables and dairy produce, all of which are heavily contaminated with pesticides and fertilizers, if inorganic produce is selected. To add to this load, inorganic animal produce is laden with hormones and antibiotics, both of which are a challenge to the detoxifying and eliminating organs – the liver and kidneys of a young child. It has been estimated that 50 per cent of the antibiotics to which a child is exposed actually come from the food he eats, rather than from antibiotics that have been prescribed.

If buying organic food is prohibitive from a cost point of view, look at reducing the amount of animal produce and supplementing the diet with vegetable-based proteins, such as pulses, grains, beans and sprouted seeds, all of which can be used in casseroles, purées and burgers to equally delicious effect (see Beany-burgers, page 138).

Liver alert!

The liver of any animal is one of the most densely packed sources of protein, in terms of nutrients. It is rich in vitamins A, B-complex, iron, chromium, copper, selenium and zinc – all of which are required for strong growth and immunity. However, as an organ of detoxification it is also the storehouse for all the pesticides and toxins from any non-organic food in your child's diet. Therefore if there is only *one* organic animal product that you buy for your child, make it liver, and you will truly be protecting her from the most abundant source of stored toxins, while giving her a food that is packed with nutrients. However, do be aware that, owing to its high content of vitamin A, liver should not be given to your child more than once every 10–14 days, from the age of about nine months.

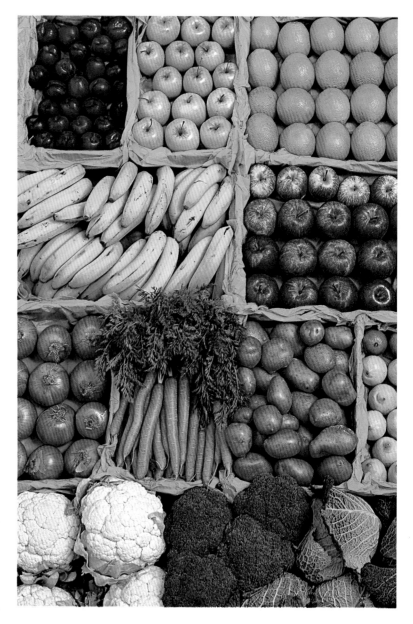

When organic isn't better

Many manufacturers have jumped on the organic bandwagon and have used the term to endorse otherwise unhealthy products. Chocolate and chocolate biscuits (organic or non-organic) are not healthy (see Sugar and spice on pages 38–41), and neither are crisps made from organically grown potatoes, if they have been deep-fried in hydrogenated fats and have had copious salt added for flavour. Beware supermarket hype: many so-called 'special' brands have been developed to seduce the unknowing buyer into believing that a product is healthier because it is organic, while simultaneously piling it with sugars and other additives. See Reading Labels (pages 42–5) for further information.

Toddler's top tip

An apple a day contains ample vitamin C, plus pectin, which binds to chemicals and pesticides, removing them safely from the body. Pears offer the same advantages, and make a tasty change.

Sugar and spice
and other things that aren't nice

How to regulate your child's glycaemic index

In order to balance the high- and low-index foods, try combining several of the foods given in the table in each meal, so that the average of all the foods chosen is on or below 50. Remember that the foods listed in the table are all mainly carbohydrate in nature, and that protein foods (from animal sources in particular) have a low glycaemic index. There are a number of books dedicated to this subject.

Porridge oats with full-fat milk and pears = 49 + 34 + 34 divided by 3 = 39

Spaghetti with tomato and sweet-potato sauce = 41 + 38 + 51 divided by 3 = 43

Baked beans on brown toast with a glass of milk = 48 + 69 + 34 divided by 3 = 50

Popcorn (unsugared) with plain yoghurt and cherries = 38 + 36 + 23 divided by 3 = 32

Baked potato with lentils, tomatoes and peas = 85 + 29 + 38 + 51 divided by 3 = 67

Sugar is found naturally in all foods, but it is also an inherent part of the Western diet, being used to flavour, enhance and preserve virtually every food product found on our supermarket shelves.

Unfortunately, excessive added sugars can have devastating repercussions on children's health, as they have a direct effect on the immune system, lowering the protection that your child needs against the abundant infections and bad bacteria that form a part of everyday life. Sugars also upset the delicate balance of beneficial bacteria found in the digestive tract, which are there to successfully digest and absorb the food your child eats.

From the first moment that a child tastes a sugar in any form, he or she will have developed an inherent liking for it, and it is therefore essential to understand which foods are beneficial and which are not.

How sugars work in the body: the glycaemic index

It is important to understand that all foods are broken down into glucose. This is then carried in the bloodstream to the muscles, brain and other organ cells, where it is converted into the energy required for the specific function of the organ in question: for example, enabling the brain to think and instruct the rest of the body to function, the lungs to breathe and the muscles to move.

Carbohydrates are the preferred source of fuel for the body as they are broken down into glucose, but proteins and fats can also be used for this purpose. For example, a piece of fish is generally recognized as being protein, but it also contains fats (known as essential fats). During the digestion process the proteins are separated from the fats, each being broken down by different enzymes at different rates of absorption. Both of these separate parts will be converted into glucose if there is no carbohydrate present in the meal. A piece of fruit, such as a banana, is essentially a carbohydrate, although it also contains a small amount of protein. Both parts will be broken down separately, but the carbohydrate section will be absorbed more rapidly than the protein (because protein takes longer to digest). Each food is thus evaluated according to the rate at which it is broken down and converted into glucose. This is known as the 'glycaemic index' of a food.

Glycaemic index of foods and drinks

Foods that have a low number on the glycaemic index release their sugars slowly and gradually. They are long-term energy-producing foods, and are more beneficial than those with a high index. You may combine some of the higher-index foods with those foods that have a lower index, to ensure a more sustained release of energy.

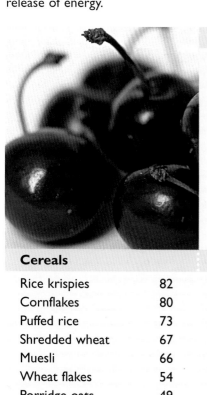

Fruits

Watermelons	72
Raisins	64
Bananas	62
Grapes	45
Oranges	40
Apples	39
Pears	34
Grapefruits	26
Plums	25
Cherries	23

Vegetables

Parsnips (cooked)	97
Carrots (cooked)	92
Potatoes (baked)	85
French fries	75
Potatoes (new)	70
Beetroots	64
Corn	59
Peas	51
Sweet potatoes	51
Tomatoes	38

Cereals

Rice krispies	82
Cornflakes	80
Puffed rice	73
Shredded wheat	67
Muesli	66
Wheat flakes	54
Porridge oats	49
Rice bran	19

Grains

White bread	95
Rice cakes	82
White rice	72
French bread	70
Brown bread	69
Crumpets	69
Brown rice	60
Pastry	59
Pitta bread	57
Oat cakes	54
Wholemeal pasta	41
Pumpernickel	40
Barley	26

Pulses

Baked beans	48
Chickpeas	36
Lima beans	36
Haricot beans	31
Kidney beans	29
Lentils	29
Soya beans	15

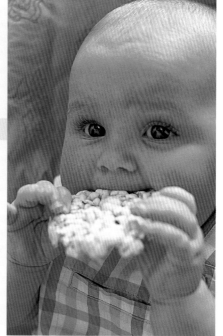

Dairy products

Ice cream	50
Plain yoghurt	36
Full-fat milk	34
Skimmed milk	32

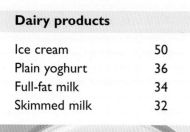

Snacks and drinks

Energy drinks	95
Jelly beans	80
Corn chips	72
Fizzy orange drink	68
Chocolate bar (milk)	68
Diluted squash	66
Orange juice	46
Apple juice	40
Popcorn	38
Dark chocolate	22

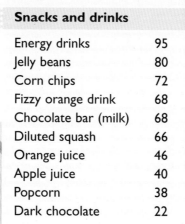

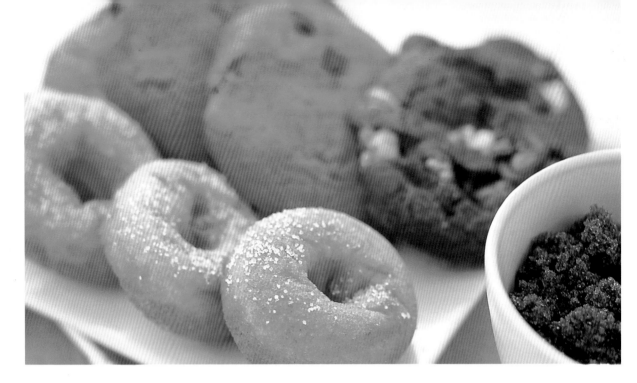

In the section on Essential building blocks (see pages 16–19) we looked at the difference between simple and complex carbohydrates. Food such as pasta – which is a refined, highly processed carbohydrate – is broken down in the digestion process and converted into glucose very rapidly, providing a short, sharp burst of energy. This food has a very high glycaemic index – that is, it will rapidly raise the level of glucose in the bloodstream and give your child an abundance of immediate energy, usually followed by a craving for something sweet, because subconsciously he or she is trying to maintain that energy 'high'. Sweet foods are often chosen at this point: packets of crisps, biscuits and commercially prepared children's puddings all contain large quantities of added sugars. This type of eating pattern can become a vicious circle, as more and more refined foods are required to keep up energy levels.

Unfortunately, there is a price to pay for this type of convenience eating, because the body cannot maintain itself with a high glucose level in the blood – and it has its own way of coping with such an event. Insulin, which is used to take glucose from the blood in circulation to the organ cells throughout the body, is dumped into the bloodstream, and your child experiences this as sudden fatigue, apathy and/or irritability.

Think of a children's tea party – all laughter until the sweets, chocolate biscuits and birthday cake arrive. Within minutes voices get raised an octave or two, and the playing turns from fun to pinching and punching; within half an hour you have a roomful of irritable, tired or destructive kids, who all need to go home before someone gets hurt! This is a prime example of fluctuating blood-glucose levels due to the child's sensitivity to refined carbohydrates and sweeteners.

It's not only cakes and biscuits that contain sugar – all fruits and vegetables contain natural sugars.

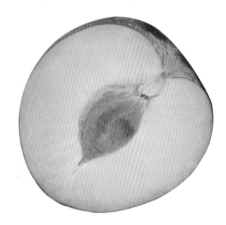

It is therefore useful to have a basic knowledge of which foods have a high glycaemic index and which have a lower index, so that you can mix the two for a more even release of energy in your child. All healthy children should have natural highs and lows during the day, but dramatic changes in mood and physical exertion can all be controlled by what your child is eating. See the table on page 39

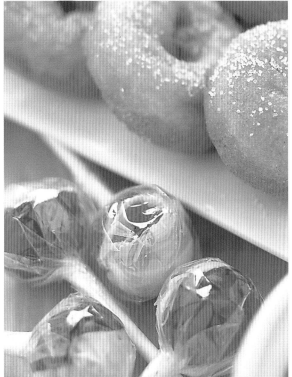

Secretive sugars

Many so-called 'healthy' foods contain sugars for flavouring or preserving. Becoming aware of these will help you to minimize their use in your meal-planning.

Food	Quantity	Sugars
Fruit yoghurt	I small carton	4 tsp
Jam	2 teaspoons	2½ tsp
Ice cream	I scoop	2 tsp
Canned sweetcorn	½ can	2 tsp
Baked beans	I small can	1½ tsp
Canned tomato soup	½ can	I tsp
Tomato ketchup	I tablespoon	I tsp
Milk chocolate	I small bar	6½ tsp
Digestive biscuits	2 biscuits	I tsp
Smarties	I tube	7½ tsp

for the 'highs' and 'lows' of the glycaemic index of specific foods.

When is a sugar natural, and when is it not?

All fruits and vegetables contain natural sugars, as do grains. The sugars in a food are actually part of the growing process, and you will have noticed that fresh young carrots, for example, are sweeter than larger, older varieties. It is the natural sugars in a food that play a role in the energy supply to your child as part of the digestion/absorption process. But remember that these are natural sugars – not added sugars. The vitamin and mineral content of these natural foods also plays an essential role in your child's diet and it is important, after the early weaning stage, to balance these naturally sweet foods with adequate proteins, which tend to have a much lower level of sugar and which slow down the process of digestion.

When a sugar has been added to a food in its preparation, it is not attached to the food itself and is therefore digested in a different way. Added sugars are digested far more rapidly, and they alter the body's natural balance of glucose in the blood. Starchy grains, such as wheat and corn, already contain abundant natural sugars, so commercial cereals that have been refined (combined with the added sugars that are used as flavour enhancers, and the dried fruits that are often included, which concentrate the sugar sources) provide an excessive amount of sugars in one meal. A bowl of porridge oats with grated apple and sliced banana is much more beneficial, and even more delicious!

Many convenience snacks and commercially prepared foods for children have excessive sugars to make them more appealing – usually in the form of coloured icings, crusty toppings or chocolate coatings. Cereals are frequently coated in honey, while sauces and ketchups are loaded with sugars, as are commercially prepared, tinned or ready-to-eat pasta dishes, particularly those with tomato-based sauces. While this may be a necessary part of preserving food to prolong its shelf-life in the suupermarket, there is little that is beneficial for your child in such foods.

Reading labels

Manufacturers have developed a huge range of label jargon, which is often confusing and sometimes even misleading. Understanding what you are reading can go a long way towards not being fooled, as well as knowing how to balance what you serve your child from a tin or packet, in addition to fresh foods.

Serving size

All ingredients are listed by serving/portion size, or per 4oz/100g. It is therefore important to know the size of the portion being served (e.g. 6oz/150g pot of yoghurt), which may then be multiplied by the amount of carbohydrates, proteins and fats per 4oz/100g in order to calculate the total.

The illustration below shows the different sections of a label that you might find on a tin, packet or pre-packed meal. There are several different areas to read, with some major points to look out for.

Check out the ingredients

According to current EU law, all ingredients that make up more than 2 per cent of a product must be listed on the packaging. The first ingredient given (e.g. 'wheat flour') constitutes the highest percentage in the product; the second ingredient (e.g. 'sugar') constitutes the next highest, and so on. Any colouring, additive, emulsifier (an agent that ensures fats are mixed into the other ingredients without separating or curdling), thickener or stabilizer must also be listed. This is where the problems often start, because many of these ingredients are listed simply by E-number.

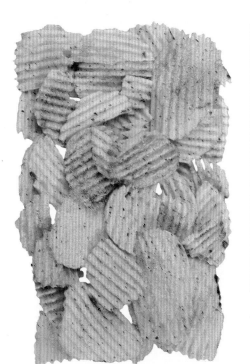

Ingredients: oats (18%), glucose syrup, crisped rice (containing rice and dried milk powder), raisins (9%), honey (8%), dried apricots (7.6%), hydrogenated vegetable oil and vegetable oil, malted wheatflakes, fructose, brown sugar, emulsifier, citric acid, flavourings, gelling agent MAY CONTAIN TRACES OF NUTS

NUTRITION INFORMATION

TYPICAL VALUES	PER BAR	PER 100G
Energy	550kJ	1574kJ
	130kcal	374kcal
PROTEIN	2.0g	5.8g
CARBOHYDRATE	26.8g	73.4g
of which sugars	12.8g	37.2g
FAT	3.2g	9.4g
Of which saturates	0.7g	2.2g
FIBRE	1.4g	4.2g
SODIUM	0.05g	0.012g

The above is an example of a typical food label for a nutrition bar.

The dreaded E-numbers

Not all E-numbers are bad! Many of them are natural ingredients, and it is well worth familiarizing yourself with those most frequently used, and those that are most damaging, so that you know at a glance which ingredients may be harmful to your child. The Foods Standards Agency (see Resources, pages 156–7) publishes a booklet on E-numbers, which is free of charge and pocket-sized, so arm yourself with this is in the first instance, in order to acquire a better knowledge of this subject.

Sugars: the 'oses'

Sucrose, maltose, dextrose, fructose, maltodextrose, glucose, lactose, mannotose, cane sugar, sugar syrup, corn syrup, hydrolized starch, inverted sugar – these are all forms of sugar, as well as 'sugar' itself of course. In children's speciality and novelty foods, which are usually laden with sugars, you may find two or more of these ingredients in one product. When you add up the sugars (see Carbohydrates, page 45), you will notice that often they constitute almost the entire carbohydrate content of a food. Remember that feeding these types of sugars to your child will only lead to cravings for more of the same. So reduce the roller-coaster ride of mood swings throughout the day by minimizing or cutting out such products from your child's diet.

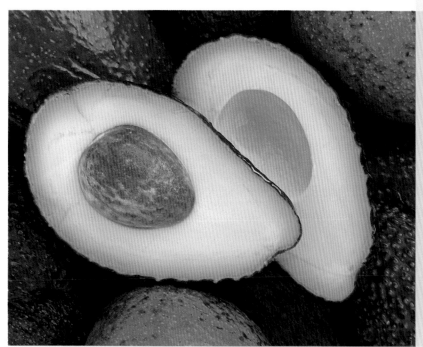

Calorie counter – measuring energy

One of the most misleading measurements of all on food packaging concerns the calorie count of a product. As adults, we seem to be constantly in search of low-calorie foods, mistakenly believing that they are low-fat foods. Not so! The kilocalorie (K-cal) was originally designed as a measurement of how much energy output could be derived from any given food, including fresh fruits and vegetables; it was never a measurement of fat content, although a food that is high in fat is also high in K-cals, since it provides a lot of energy.

Take the avocado, which is often viewed as a 'fattening' food, offering 300–500 calories per avocado. In fact it is so high in calories because you can derive much energy from this one simple food, while its fat content is actually made up of beneficial omega-6 essential fats, which are required for hormone and brain development in children, as well as B vitamins for energy. So an avocado is probably one of the most energy-packed snacks you can give your child.

Too much/too little

The British Heart Foundation has produced a chart that makes reading labels straightforward and simple. It lists the amount of fat and other ingredients in a product that would be considered a small amount, and the amount that would be considered too much.

Too much	A little
20g fat	3g fat
5g saturates	1g saturates
10g sugar	2g sugar
0.5g sodium	0.1g sodium

A typical sweet snack (such as a chocolate-chip cookie) includes a high level of sugar, fat and saturates, as well as a moderate-to-high level of sodium. Sodium, or salt, is used to stabilize products such as ketchups, sauces and tinned foods so that they have a longer shelf-life. Sugar is also used as a stabilizer for long-life products, and particularly for fresh dairy foods such as fruit yoghurts. (For more on sugars and where they may be hidden, see Sugar and spice, pages 38–41.)

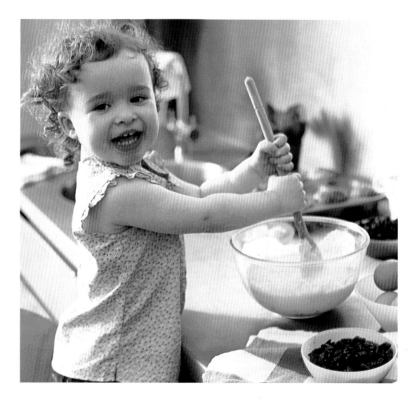

The fat story

As we have already seen, fats are broken down into various categories:

- Saturated: fats that originate from an animal source – often considered to be the most 'fatty' of all the fats. They provide your child with healthy fats only when they are not deep-fried (e.g. bacon bits and oven chips).
- Unsaturated: fats that are found in vegetarian sources of protein, such as nuts, seeds and their oils. Olive oil, for example, is a mono-unsaturated fat and is perfectly healthy. Pumpkin seeds are poly-unsaturated fats (being primarily omega-6) and are both healthy and beneficial.

When looking at the fat content of any food, you therefore need to look closely to see what percentage of the total product is fat, and whether there is a high level of sodium in the product, which would indicate that the product has been fried in its preparation, or that it needs to be heated to a high temperature to serve (which will kill all the beneficial nutrients in the food).

Remember that if a food is of animal protein origin, it will inherently have a relatively high level of fat, which is acceptable provided that you are not serving other foods with the main dish that contain equally high levels of fat (such as a pudding that is rich in dairy products). It is the combination of too much fat at one meal that overloads your child's digestive system and may lead to weight gain in the long term.

Carbohydrates

The carbohydrates in a product will always be listed after the protein content, and will be separated into the total carbohydrates (e.g. oats in porridge) and a subheading entitled 'of which sugars'. It is important to check this latter category, as it will give you a very clear indication of what percentage the sugars form in the whole product. For example, an apparently healthy muesli bar might contain 65.5 per cent carbohydrates per 4oz/100g, of which 49 per cent is sugar. Therefore nearly a third of the muesli bar that your child is eating actually consists of sugar!

Becoming familiar with label reading is not difficult, once you know how to approach it, and forms an important part of managing your child's food consumption.

Toddler's top tip
Giving your child fresh raw vegetables, such as carrots, celery, apples and pears, as snacks reduces the number of packet alternatives that are high in additives and colourants.

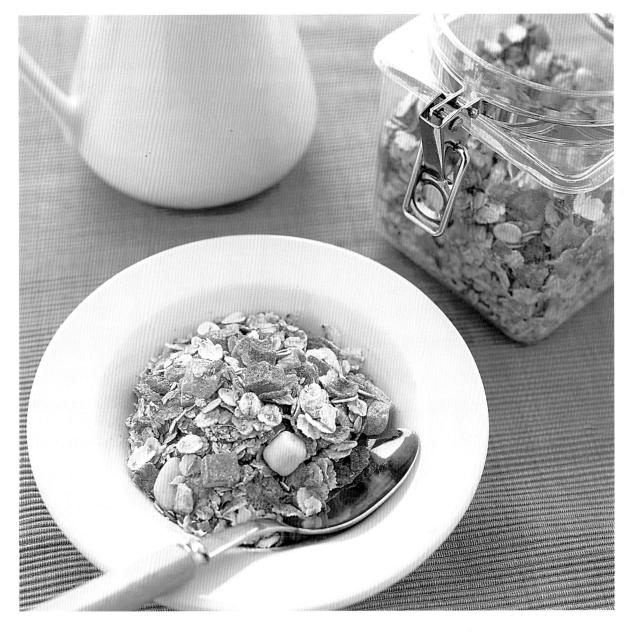

The storage cupboard

Having a well-stocked larder is the sign of a well-prepared kitchen (not of a lazy cook!). Being organized offers some relief from having to prepare fresh food daily, and lets you relax when nipping out to the supermarket becomes an impossibility, for example when one of the children is sick and you can't leave home.

Tins of beans and lentils and tomato sauces represent an efficient way of having plenty of mixers that take no time to prepare – and very few of us now have the time to soak beans overnight, then boil them twice, prior to using these highly nutritious foods in our children's dishes. Many of these foods keep their nutritional value if they are combined creatively with fresh produce (such as chicken, eggs and vegetables) in casseroles and soups.

Use the following list as a reminder that you carry with you whenever you are in the supermarket – in this way you will never be caught short of something nutritious to serve your child.

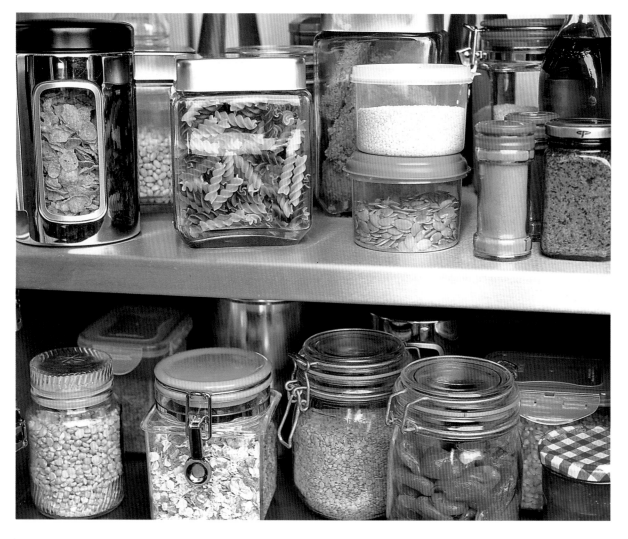

Storage-cupboard shopping list

Dry goods
Wholegrain brown basmati rice
Buckwheat pasta or orzo
Corn pasta
Wholegrain spaghetti or
   tagliatelle
Polenta (corn/maize meal)
Barley
Millet flakes
Couscous
Bulgur wheat

Cereals and biscuits
Jumbo oats for porridge
Muesli mix
Cornflakes (unsweetened)
Rice puffs (unsweetened)
Ryvita
Rye crackers
Water biscuits
Oat cakes
Rice crackers

Dried fruits
Apricots
Raisins
Prunes
Figs
Peaches
Mango
Apple rings

Pulses (tinned or dried)
Lentils
Yellow split peas
Kidney beans
Black-eyed beans
Chickpeas
Butterbeans

Jams/spices/herbs/sauces/ oils and vinegars
Low-sugar jam/marmalade
Nutmeg
Cinnamon
Vanilla pod (a natural sweetener)
Star anise
Powdered ginger
Dried basil, sage and rosemary
Mango chutney
Tomato purée
Low-sugar ketchup (can be
   home-made)
Pesto sauce
Tamari sauce (wheat-free soy
   sauce)
Olive oil
Walnut oil
Sunflower oil
Sesame oil
Wine vinegar
Apple cider vinegar
Lemon juice

Tinned foods
Sardines
Tuna
Salmon
Organic (low-sugar) baked beans
Chopped tomatoes
Cherries
Pears
Apricots

Baby foods
Dry formula-milk preparations
Tins or jars of vegetables and
   fruits (preferably organic)
Rusks (low-sugar varieties only)

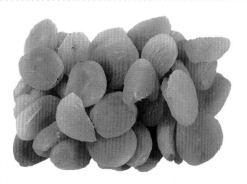

Make sure that you do not rely on these foods and flavourings as the mainstay of your child's diet; instead, use them to complement fresh foods bought daily. There is no substitute for serving fresh fruit and vegetables, although many tinned foods (such as fish) do adequately preserve their nutrient content and ensure that your child is getting the protein she needs for growth.

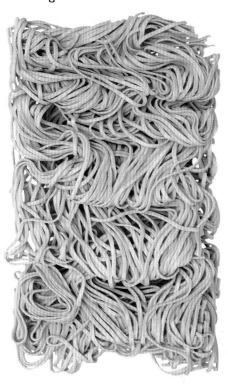

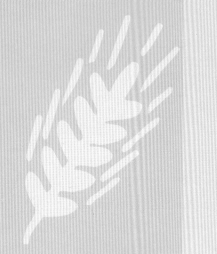

Eating habits and special diets

Children are inherently aware of what foods do and don't suit them. They allow their noses and tongues to be their guides, and will often turn away from foods that are likely to cause some kind of reaction.

Providing good choice and variety from an early age is key to reducing the likelihood of a child developing allergies or sensitivities. In fact, most children have few (if any) specific food sensitivities.

Some children will eat everything put in front of them; others are more fussy, or seek certain foods for specific reasons. Understanding the possible contributory factors in refusing to eat may well reduce hours of frustration and wasted cooking time. The following section aims to shed more light on these specific dietary needs and habits.

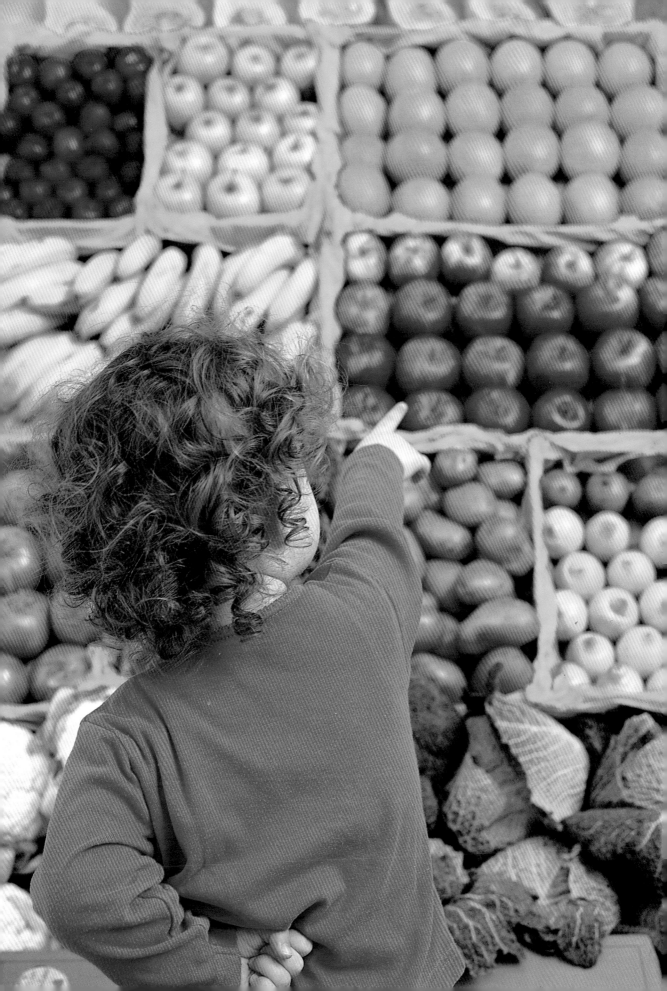

When your child won't eat

Physical reasons for refusing to eat

1. Your child is unwell: it is natural for children to refuse food when they are developing an ailment. Many parents take loss of appetite as an early warning sign. Make sure he has plenty of fluids to prevent dehydration, and include a mineral-salts solution (such as Dioralyte), if he has developed diarrhoea, to prevent the possibility of mineral imbalances.

2. Physical inactivity: if your child has not been running around all day, but has been sitting in front of the television, she will not have burned up as much energy as if she had spent the afternoon on the playing fields. Gauge your child's appetite from her specific energy requirements.

3. The food is off: children's tastebuds are usually more sensitive than those of adults, and they will detect if something on their plate is not going to sit well in their tummy!

4. Teething, or growing second sets of teeth, will cause genuine discomfort when eating: check that your child's teeth are coming through correctly, and that there isn't a problem with overcrowding.

There are times when your child's eating habits appear to change overnight – having been an unfussy eater, and apparently loving his food, he may suddenly appear disinterested, moody or simply 'not hungry'. There are several very real reasons for this – not necessarily just 'playing up'.

The issue of control is a major one when it comes to food: your child may elicit the most radical reaction from you by refusing to eat, and this may leave you feeling frustrated and angry especially when you have spent time preparing a fresh meal with good intentions. He will see that he has managed to get a reaction from you and may try to use this to manipulate you in the future. This isn't bad behaviour – it is simply your child testing his boundaries and using his intellect!

It is important not to apply pressure at such a time as this can lead, in the long term, to eating issues and hidden behaviour. Instead, try to talk to him about why he doesn't want to eat. Give him the opportunity to express himself, rather than punishing him with threats of 'If you don't eat your main course, you won't get a pudding'. Many children are forced to eat foods that ultimately do not suit their digestion, so it is important not to ignore stomach cramps and diarrhoea, which are very real symptoms of intolerance that usually appear before your child's voice makes itself heard. Conversely, children who have a tendency to vomit after or during eating may be exhibiting early signs of an eating disorder (see Overweight or underweight on pages 52–3).

Eating together

Many working families and parents often miss their children's mealtimes, arriving home after they have finished eating. Try to arrange your schedule so that you can have at least one meal a day with your children, and encourage this to be a time to enjoy food and conversation together. There is no reason why you shouldn't all be eating much the same food together and, with different-aged children, the younger ones may be invited to try the more grown-up meals, to eliminate any feeling of being left out. Assume that your child may want to try anything, and that no food is 'for adults only', unless there is a problem with a known intolerance.

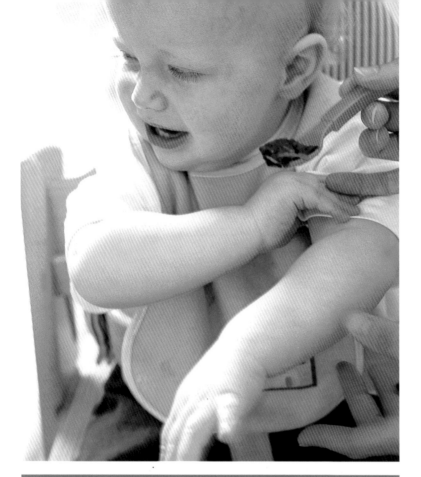

Top tips for no-fuss eating

Serve small portions: your child can have a second helping.

Introduce new foods one at a time: no child is happy with a completely new arrangement of foods on their plate that they do not recognize.

Make mealtimes fun and relaxed: sit and chat together, rather than rushing through the meal, but don't allow your child to play with toys at the table – he will use them as a distraction.

Ensure that the plate of food is colourful and attractive: you wouldn't want to be faced with overcooked, bland-coloured food, any more than your child does.

Don't get angry with your child when he won't eat. Ask him what the problem is, and encourage him to talk.

Provide regular snacks between meals to keep blood-sugar levels balanced such as fresh fruit and raw vegetables, or small pieces of cheese and crackers.

Irritability is a sign of hunger. Plan your mealtimes to avoid such extremes, as he is less likely to eat if he is over-hungry or tired.

Let your child participate in the preparation of meals: most children are fascinated by the process of putting meals together.

Emotional reasons for refusing to eat

1. Concern over weight: children are becoming aware of their bodies at a disconcertingly young age nowadays. It is not uncommon for girls aged seven or eight to be talking about dieting and the way they look in their clothes. If you have had a weight issue yourself, try to ensure that you don't impress this attitude on your child too early. It is perfectly healthy for a child up to the age of 10 or 11 to have puppy fat on her arms or legs; equally, some children are tall and very lean, and may be self-conscious of their appearance when having to change clothes in front of their peers at school. Open conversation is the best way forward – being judgemental may only exacerbate the problem.

2. Fear of something: your child may be trying to tell you something else and using 'not hungry' as an attention ploy. While children tend to do this as part of game-playing, it is worth spending time checking on her real motivation, particularly if she suddenly stops eating properly at school. Is she being bullied, or might she be struggling in one class or another? All children lose their appetite when they are fearful.

Overweight or underweight

There is great concern about obesity among children, since the research indicates a steady increase in childhood obesity every year; and much has been written about the lack of physical activity among children, compared with 15 or 20 years ago.

Reasons for being overweight

- Eating to deal with stress or unhappiness
- Eating too many highly sugared foods, or those with a high glycaemic index (see pages 38–41)
- Eating too much at each meal
- Drinking excessive amounts of highly sugared drinks
- Not getting enough exercise
- Eating too many snacks between meals
- Hormonal disruption, specifically of the thyroid gland (a medical condition that requires diagnosis by a doctor or other health-care practitioner)
- Insufficient absorption of key nutrients, which will make your child feel 'hungry all the time' – look at the amount of 'empty' calories he may be eating.

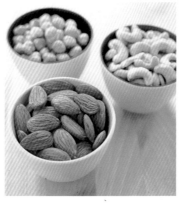

Too much, too big to handle

The reality is staggering – the number of children developing obesity has doubled in the last 20 years in the USA, and the figure is not much lower in the UK, with nearly one-third of all children being clinically obese by the age of 11. While much of this may be due to a lower rate of physical activity and a much greater number of hours spent in front of the television, in truth we have to look at the foods we are now giving our children. When we examine the vast number of convenience snacks that are available to 'keep children quiet', it is little wonder that the pounds creep on.

It is known that children lay down their fat cells in the first five years of life and, once there, they are difficult to shift. It is a great disadvantage to any child to have to face a life of inhibited or restricted eating habits to curtail those little fat cells' greed! However, it should be understood that the family environment plays a large part in the weight game, and the child of two heavy parents is more likely to be heavy himself.

Light as a feather

Being underweight is a different type of problem altogether, but one that can lead to equal anxiety for your child. There are many reasons for a child being thin, most of which are metabolic and physical. She may well have a seemingly insatiable appetite, and be described as being able to 'eat like a horse' without putting on a pound! There is no harm in this, and care should be taken to ensure that she is able to eat regularly to keep her blood-sugar levels balanced.

But it is also important to be aware of a potential underlying emotional component in wanting to 'look cool', or of your child being aware of current trends in dieting and the desire to look like models, actors or other image-influential stars.

Such behaviour can lead to restricted eating, or opting for a 'healthy' diet: deciding to become vegetarian, or eating only large quantities of fruits, salads and vegetables, and steering clear of grains, meats and poultry, on grounds that are not always clearly defined. The age for this type of behaviour has lowered from the early teens to as young as seven or eight in girls in particular, and care should be taken to ensure that they are not skipping meals when at school or away from home.

Whilst there is much hype about the influences on a young child's self-image from the press, films and television, there is also a nutritional aspect that should not be overlooked. Some children use up far more proteins and more of the mineral zinc in their development and growth, or tend to favour a diet that is high in carbohydrates (such as pasta, bread and rice), making their diet inherently low in zinc.

Zinc has been found to be almost completely deficient in children and teenagers who are suffering from anorexia, bulimia and other eating disorders, and is intricately connected to the brain cells that govern self-image and self-esteem. Offering pre-digested proteins and zinc in the form of nutritional supplementation can arrest the development of a more serious long-term problem, but this approach should only be considered on the advice of a nutrition consultant or other health-care practitioner.

The responsibility has to lie initially with the parent to check the balance and healthiness of food choices. Often a child will start to eat in an uncontrollable fashion once his weight has started to escalate, as he doesn't understand what to do. Work out a programme with a nutrition consultant or other health-care practitioner if you are unsure what food choices are right for your child.

Toddler's top tip

Offer your child healthy nibbles, such as raw vegetables, dips and fresh fruit, for in-between meal snacks, rather than salty or sweet convenience foods.

A more serious problem

The development of a serious eating disorder can, and does, happen very rapidly, and the underlying reasons are not always immediately apparent. The management of anorexia or bulimia in a child of any age needs to be handled by professional therapists and nutrition consultants or dieticians, for the cost to the development of a child's body and hormonal balance can be devastating. Many such children are found to exist literally on cola drinks and a little fruit, on a daily basis for months at a time, while periodically bingeing to temporarily satisfy a starving body. Do not ignore signs that lead you to suspect there may be a problem – by the time you have noticed them, it may well have been developing for many months. See Resources (pages 156–7) for organizations that can help you find suitable practitioners to advise you on this area of your child's health.

Reasons for being underweight

- Nutritional deficiencies
- Loss of appetite
- Burning food at a rapid rate
- Poor absorption of nutrients from food
- Restricted eating
- Inappropriate/imbalanced vegetarianism
- Emotional imbalances
- Manipulating parents or people around them

Changing needs

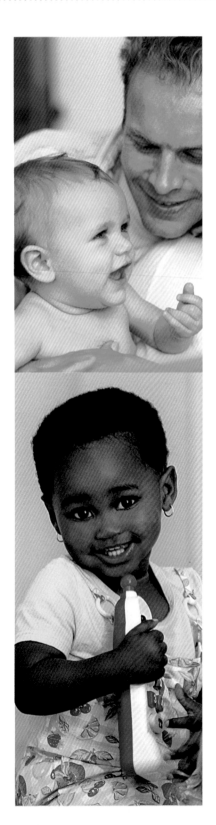

How many times have you heard a parent complain that her child will only eat pasta and potatoes? Or that she won't eat any vegetables, and will eat chicken, but not eggs?

Some children may well be fussy eaters, but this kind of complaint usually relates to a stage of your child's growth, either physically or mentally, and it is worth looking at what stage she has reached to determine what are the best types of food at this time. In Part 2 we shall explore which specific foods are needed for various stages of growth, but it is important to understand those foods that provide different sources of nutrients for your child at any given time.

The pasta/potato syndrome

As carbohydrates, pasta and potatoes provide one of the most readily available forms of energy for your child. Given the choice, he may always primarily select these foods, and refuse or turn down meat and poultry in favour of pasta or chips. If so, it is important to ensure some protein on his plate to provide for growth and development. But perhaps the main question to be asked is: 'How much energy does your child need now?'

If your child has just started to learn to walk or talk, or has just begun school, started a sport or physical activity, he may suddenly develop a ravenous appetite and seem able to consume large quantities of food. The type of food that will give him the greatest energy in the shortest time is carbohydrates, in the form of grain-based cereals, pasta or starches such as potatoes. Although these foods have a relatively high glycaemic index (see Sugar and spice, pages 38–41), they provide instant energy and an uplifted mood, and your child responds to that.

Serotonin: the happy factor

The brain contains two main neurotransmitter chemicals – serotonin and dopamine. Serotonin is known to produce feelings of well-being, excitement and laughter, while dopamine tends to cause relaxation, calm and quietness (including sleep). In balance, these two chemicals sit at opposite ends of the seesaw, regulating your child's mood from moment to moment. However, several foods and drinks can upset this delicate harmony, and this is one of the main causes of hyperactivity – when it is chemically induced (see Recognizing hyperactivity, pages 70–71).

Interestingly, carbohydrates eaten on their own will noticeably raise levels of serotonin within a short space of time, and children often become sensitive to this, without understanding why. This is a different effect from that created by your child eating a packet of crisps, a couple of biscuits or a bar of chocolate; this latter effect is more pronounced, and it is likely to be the sugars that are inducing a mild level of over-activity, rather than the carbohydrates creating a quick source of energy.

Either way, the best thing for your child is to include some form of protein (in animal or vegetable form) to create a balance and to ensure that he maintains his energy levels, and happy mood, over a longer period of time. For instance, include some walnut oil in the pasta; make some pesto sauce (using pine nuts); or add diced ham or chicken to a tomato sauce, so that the protein content is not as obvious as having to eat an entire chicken breast.

All legs and arms

The speed of growth that children experience at this stage necessitates different nutrients in varying ratios for bones, muscles and skin. While it is well-known that calcium is required for bone development throughout a child's life, the other nutrients that enable calcium to be absorbed into bone tissue are equally important – these include magnesium, boron, manganese and vitamin D. Calcium is found in all dairy produce, but not all children are tolerant of everyday food products, so awareness of other sources helps to ensure that your child is obtaining the optimum from his diet. Non-dairy sources of calcium include sardines, salmon, egg yolks, broccoli, sesame, pumpkin and sunflower seeds, and almonds and walnuts. In addition, green leafy vegetables will provide adequate magnesium to work with the calcium, enabling healthy growth of bones and teeth.

Allowing Change

Although it is frustrating to have to adapt to your child's changing needs, remember that this happens for biological reasons, rather than just because your child is changing his mind. Fussy eating is a separate issue, but it is perfectly normal for your child to love a food one week and loathe it the next. Ideally, don't stock large quantities of any one kind of food, as you may be stuck with it later!

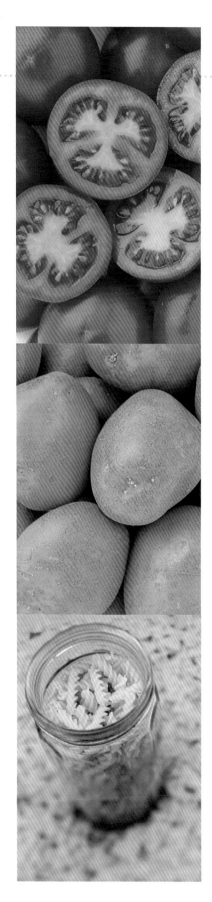

Red/orange/yellow vegetables and fruits

Carrots
Pumpkin
Sweet potatoes
Squash
Parsnip
Swede
Red/orange/yellow peppers
Tomatoes
Pomegranates
Red apples
Pears
Blackberries
Raspberries
Strawberries
Cherries
Watermelon
Apricots
Mango
Oranges
Plums
Peaches
Papaya

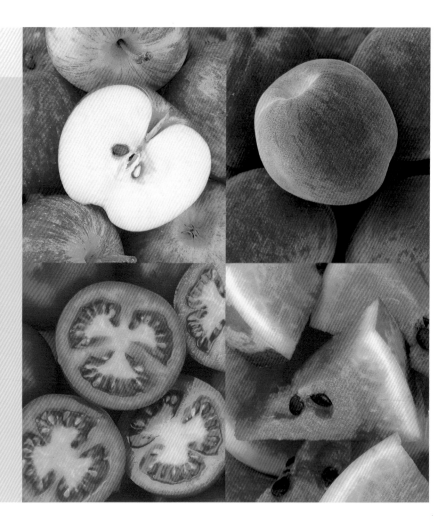

No greens today, thank you

The endless frustration of trying to make your child eat vegetables is a common one for many parents and is not always easy to overcome. Attempting to hide vegetables in tomato-based sauces is not necessarily the best approach, because if your child finds out, she may be suspicious of every new food that you put in front of her in future. The best way to approach the 'no greens' problem is to go for another colour instead! Although green vegetables contain the broadest vitamin and mineral content of all, providing other groups of vegetables (and fruits) will at least ensure that a large part of her nutritional requirements are met on a daily basis. Supplementing with a liquid multi-vitamin may also be helpful (see Vitamin and mineral requirements, pages 152–5).

Many vegetables and fruits can be juiced together to create a vitamin-rich concoction (see box above). Smoothies and puddings can also be made by combining some of the puréed fruits with plain bio-yoghurt or custard (see Puddings and treats, pages 144–7).

Vegetables may be puréed and coated with breadcrumbs to create croquettes, and then shallow-fried; these take little time to prepare, may be frozen in batches, and offer an excellent way of ensuring a wide variety of nutrients. Root vegetables tend to have sufficient natural sweetness to tempt even the most discerning palate!

Remember that many children will not eat cooked vegetables, but they will be quite happy to munch on the raw varieties. So make sure you have a supply of carrot sticks, courgette batons and celery sticks in the fridge, to offer as a fresh snack prior to giving them anything from a packet. Nowadays most supermarkets supply trays of ready-prepared crudités to make life simpler for you – include some of these in your child's lunch box, instead of chocolate biscuits.

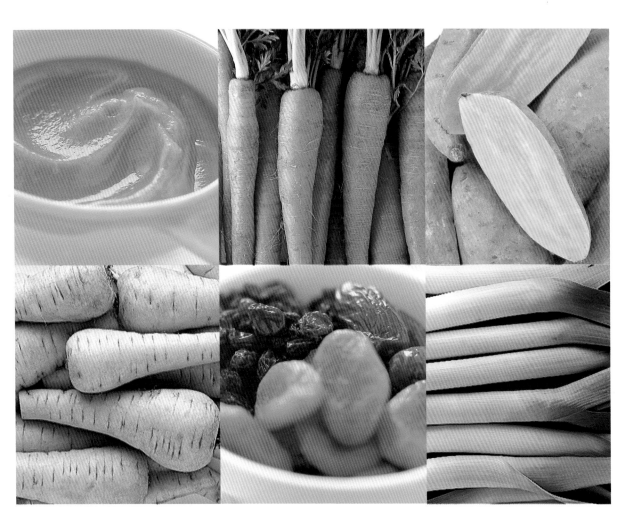

Soups also offer an opportunity to include many vegetables, such as parsnips, leeks, carrots and sweet potato (all of which help to thicken the soup, and may be puréed). Adding apricots or raisins to puddings to sweeten the taste naturally also provides a source of iron, which may be in short supply in your child's diet if he is eating few greens.

Hidden iron

Remember that a lack of iron is not the only cause of anaemia. Vitamin B6, folate and vitamin B12 are also required in regular supply to ensure the production of red blood cells. Both these nutrients are found in all animal meats and proteins, as well as wholegrains such as barley, millet, rye and oats. Thus a bowl of porridge with milk, and fresh peaches or figs, raisins or sultanas makes for a good start to the day.

Whatever food fad your child appears to have at any given time, a diet that is varied will prevent any serious nutritional deficiencies from occurring in the long term. Discipline and not taking 'No' for an answer are important, but not to the point of force-feeding. Remember to make the kitchen – and the dinner table – a friendly, fun place to be.

Iron-rich foods
- Watercress
- Egg yolks
- Oatmeal (porridge)
- Brown rice
- Lentils
- Apricots
- Raisins/sultanas
- Peaches
- Figs

Food for comfort

From the moment of birth, suckling is a natural reflex for a baby seeking the comfort and nourishment of its mother's nipple. It is inevitable that this reflex continues long after weaning from the breast has taken place.

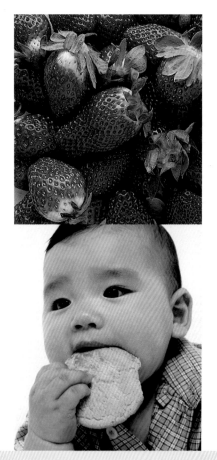

There are several schools of thought about the advisability of using dummies (pacifiers) to calm an upset baby, and the jury is still out over whether or not they should be used for more than a few weeks after weaning, because in the long term they can cause damage to teeth alignment. Many infants also become very attached to their cuddly toys and to the soft blankets in their cots and beds, and this is understood to represent comfort as well.

It is small wonder, then, that food can satisfy the same reflex, and that many children enjoy sucking on solid foods (which tend to be sweet) for extended periods of time while engaging in other activities, such as watching television or playing with dolls.

Understanding the role that the sucking reflex plays in your child's sense of security will allow you to determine when and where such behaviour might be appropriate. Conversely, children often want to have a sweet lollipop or ice-cream purely for its sugar content, and not because they need a security prop. If security is what your child is seeking, then holding her hand, or picking her up to cuddle her, may well be more appropriate.

Denying your child personal comfort is ultimately more neglectful than denying her food at the right time! Talking to and reassuring her in the first instance is preferable to simply offering her a food substitute, as this latter option may lead to manipulative behaviour with food choices later on.

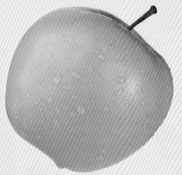

A sweet tooth?

Warm foods are most satisfying to an infant, because breast milk is at body temperature and warm food is easier to swallow than cold. From the age of about three or four, children become less particular about the temperature of their food and more conscious of taste. From the first sweet food that a child tastes, she will retain a memory of that taste, although it is not yet known what distinguishes a child who has a sweet tooth from one who doesn't.

It is safe to assume that foods that are naturally sweet, such as root vegetables and fruits, are less likely to cause sugar cravings than foods

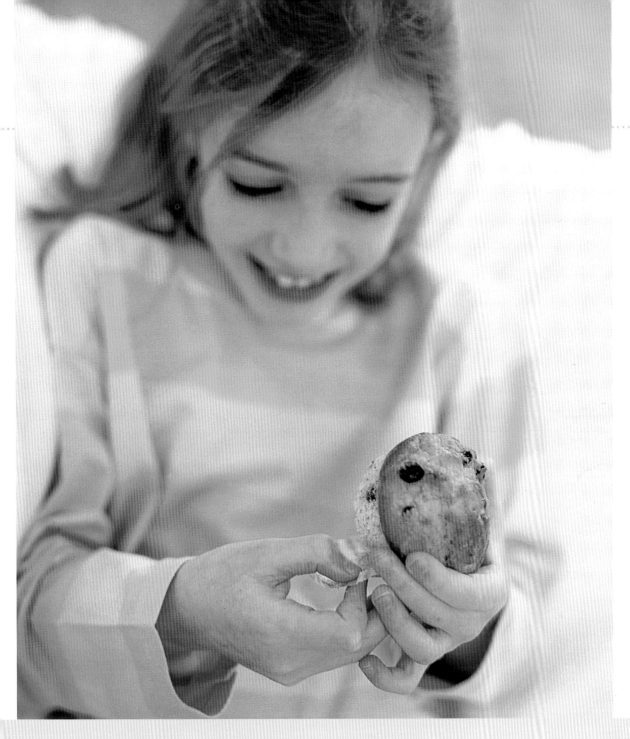

that have been artificially sweetened. This is why giving your child puddings derived mainly from fruits to satisfy his craving for something sweet (rather than chocolates, toffees or other highly sugared foods) is infinitely preferable. Making sure that there is always plenty of fresh fruit available to eat at any time of the day sends a straightforward healthy message to your child. And suggesting that she has a piece of fruit prior to eating anything that is unnaturally sweetened will often curb the desire for large quantities of sweets and confectionery later in life. When collecting your child from school, offer her a piece of fruit, rather than a chocolate bar, to provide her with a healthier pick-up.

Food for reward

It is natural for a child to consistently seek his parents' love and approval, and one of the ways to measure this achievement is through reward. How many times have you heard a child say, 'If I do such-and-such, can I have so-and-so?' This type of bartering is learned from the parents in the first place, so it is important to look at how food is used as a reward – either at the family table or right away from the kitchen.

Typical situations in which food is used as a reward:

- Clean your room/playroom, and then you can have an ice-cream.
- Finish your main course, then I shall let you have some pudding.
- Go and play quietly for the next half hour, and then you can have a chocolate.
- Do your homework and then you can have a biscuit.

Whatever the situation, the message that is coming across is one of using sweet foods as a reward (rather than an apple, a banana or carrot sticks, which are unlikely to elicit the same level of enthusiasm).

Food as nourishment, not punishment

What is perhaps more important is to look at when food is being used as part of a bribe and when it is genuinely being used as a treat because your child deserves it. Children should learn that *all* natural food is good, and that no food is ever given as a punishment – food is put on the table to nourish and feed, and not as a penance. The image of repulsive hot gruel being slapped down on the table, as shown in the gruesome meal-scenes in the film *Oliver!*, create lasting memories of food as punishment.

Perhaps the greatest danger in using food for reward inappropriately is in encouraging your child to develop an unnaturally sweet tooth, which she then has to cope with for life. Many adults in middle age have battled with obesity for a large part of their lives, having been allowed a considerable quantity of sweet foods early on.

With the growing concern about childhood obesity, and the increased risk of developing diabetes later in life because of such eating habits, it is vital that commercially sweetened foods, snacks and salted vegetable crisps should be kept to a minimum. These foods all contain chemicals that may create cravings for more of the same within a very short time. Such foods also inhibit the sensitivity of the taste-buds to the subtle nuances of natural foods. Creating delicious puddings and healthy bars and biscuits, such as grainy granola bars, adapted from the recipe for Brainy Seed Granola Cereal (see page 135), will go a long way towards avoiding such problems.

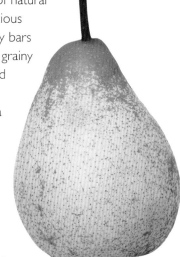

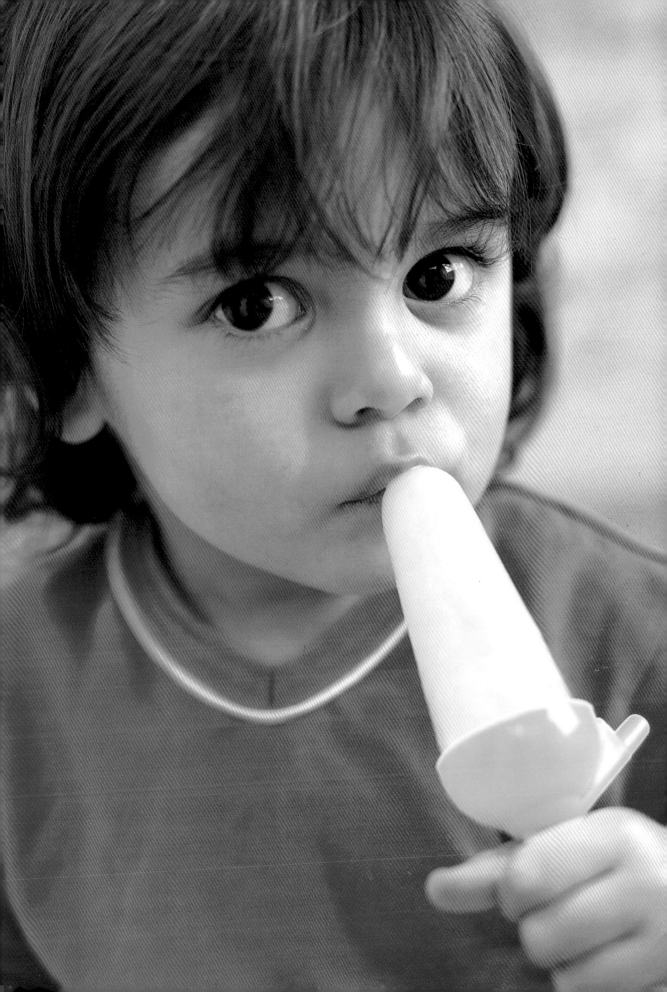

The vegetarian child

Whether or not you elect to raise your child as a vegetarian is up to you, but if you have chosen the vegetarian option, it is important to have a full understanding of which vegetable proteins will offer your child everything he needs for optimal (and not merely adequate) growth.

'There is more calcium in a serving of fresh broccoli than in a glass of milk.'
Food Values

Some children tend towards vegetarianism because they don't like the taste or texture of meat and poultry. It is important not to force any food on a child, but to look at how you can ensure that the essential nutrients will be consumed in other foods, without creating an issue for your child.

The most important nutrients found in dairy products, meat and fish are the minerals, including zinc, calcium and magnesium, iron and selenium. While calcium, magnesium and iron are all required for building healthy bones and a sound cardiovascular system, zinc and selenium are vital for healthy digestive and immune systems. It is recommended that vegetarian children take supplementary vitamin and mineral complexes every day.

Vegetable alternatives to essential minerals

	Animal source	Vegetable source
Calcium	Dairy produce, sardines, salmon	Soya beans, sunflower seeds, almonds, sesame seeds, green leafy vegetables, including broccoli
Magnesium	Crab, chicken	Dark-green leafy vegetables, lemons, grapefruits, almonds, figs, raisins, aubergines, onions, carrots, potatoes, corn
Iron	Red meat, liver, egg yolks	Nuts, sunflower seeds, millet, oatmeal, brown rice, figs, avocados, cherries, bananas, raisins, prunes, apricots, broccoli, asparagus, kale, lentils
Zinc	Meat, eggs, chicken, sardines, tuna	Sunflower seeds, pumpkin seeds, wheatgerm, buckwheat, rye, brown rice, oats, almonds, cucumbers, carrots, cauliflower, lettuce, berries
Selenium	Shellfish, seafood	Sesame seeds, wheatgerm, tomatoes, broccoli

Protein bricks

The other significant way to ensure your vegetarian child has a balanced diet is to understand how to combine vegetable-based proteins. As proteins form the building bricks of your child's body (particularly hormones, immune and digestive systems), it is vital to include as many vegetable proteins as possible, to guarantee complete protein in her diet.

Animal-based proteins are inherently 'complete' – that is, they all contain the eight essential amino acids that the body requires to create the building blocks. However, vegetable-based proteins (with the exception of soya products and seaweed, which rarely form a large part of any child's diet) are incomplete, and it is therefore necessary to combine them to provide all the amino acids on a daily basis (see Essential building blocks, pages 16–19).

The vegan issue

A vegan diet is one that contains strictly no animal protein at all. Although rare as a dietary choice for a child, it is important to understand that there is a risk of vitamin B12 deficiency in children who eat no animal produce, as this vitamin is not found in vegetable sources other than spirulina (a form of algae). In fact, it is not known whether animal or vegetable sources of vitamin B12 are actually bio-available to a child or not, and the symptoms of B12 deficiency are similar to those of iron deficiency, so taking an iron supplement may not be the answer. Choosing a vegan diet for a child is normally only an option for moral or religious reasons, and should be done with the help of a professional nutritionist or other medical expert.

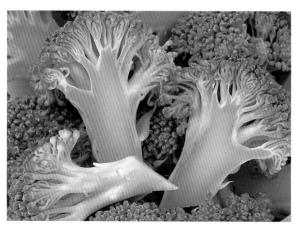

Vegetable-protein groups

So your child has a combination of amino acids, choose foods from each of the following groups.

Soya products
Miso (fermented soya-bean paste)
Tempeh (soya 'meat' alternative)
Tamari (wheat-free soy sauce)
Tofu (bean curd)

Pulses
Lentils
Split peas
Green peas

Legumes
Kidney beans
Chickpeas
Butter beans
Black-eyed beans
Garbanzo beans (used for baked beans)

Nuts and seeds
Almonds
Brazils
Walnuts
Hazelnuts
Pine nuts
Pecans
Cashews
Peanuts (check allergy risk)
Sesame
Sunflower
Pumpkin
Linseed (flaxseed)
Note: all nuts can also be used as nut butters for children who have no allergy risk

As sesame, pumpkin and sunflower seeds are difficult to break down and digest, it may be advisable to grind them and add them to soya milk and puddings to increase the protein blocks. Nuts may be added to stir-fries and casseroles for added taste as well as protein, and beans give a 'meaty' texture to soups, vegetarian burgers and rissoles.

Allergies and intolerances

It has been estimated that by the year 2005, one in every two children will experience some form of allergic reaction to food within the first 10 years of life. This may largely be due to the massive increase in additives, colourings and excipients that are now frequently added to foods to lengthen their shelf life, or make them more appealing to a child's eye.

Recognizing an acute allergy

- Facial flushing
- Shortness of breath
- Diarrhoea
- Itching mouth or lips
- Rashes (anywhere on the body)
- Abdominal pain (acute)
- Swollen lips, eyes, ears or tongue
- Fainting
- Rapid heartbeat

Recognizing a food intolerance or delayed reaction

- Colic
- Eczema
- Urticaria (hives or nettle-rash)
- Headaches
- Migraines
- Hyperactivity
- Insomnia
- Mouth ulcers
- Late bedwetting
- Continuous diarrhoea
- Glue ear (otitis media)
- Runny nose

Acute allergy or delayed food reaction?

Determining the difference between an acute allergic reaction and that of a delayed food reaction is a complicated and intricate subject, and going into full detail would provide enough text for an entire book on the subject. The easiest way to look at the difference between the two is to say that 'an acute allergic reaction is a sudden reaction to an otherwise harmless food that involves a specific part of the immune army known as IgE antibodies, that can provoke a potentially fatal series of reactions'. This is also known as 'immediate hypersensitivity', and can occur at any age.

A delayed food reaction, on the other hand, does not involve antibody reactions as such, but triggers reactions by another part of the immune army known as T-lymphocytes. As such reactions are usually not immediate, for example lactose or gluten intolerance, it makes the offending food or foods more difficult to determine.

What to do . . .

The simplest way to determine specific foods that may be causing delayed food reactions is to keep a food diary for two to three weeks to evaluate which foods are coinciding with a reaction. It may be necessary to look back as much as 48–72 hours prior to the onset of a symptom, as intolerances usually aren't immediate. Upon finding a suspect food, remove it entirely from your child's diet for two to three months (and possibly longer) before re-introducing it with caution. This will allow that part of the immune system that has previously been reacting to settle down.

In an emergency . . .

If the reaction is very acute – for instance, shortness of breath, swollen lips, eyes or tongue, or immediate vomiting – ensure that there is no obstruction in the air passageways, and that all tight clothing is loosened or removed. Keep calm and make sure that your child does not become over-excited. Take her to a doctor or hospital immediately.

Once the problem food has been identified, it must be stringently avoided for several years, and in some cases for life. Initially, this will require considerable diligence and effort, because all food labels will need to be read and understood. However, there are a large number of allergy-free alternatives on the market today.

Top 10 problem foods

1. Cow's milk
2. Dairy products
3. Wheat (and other gluten grains: rye, barley and oats)
4. Fish and shellfish
5. Citrus fruits (particularly oranges)
6. Tomatoes
7. Eggs (yolks and/or whites)
8. Soya milk and related products
9. Nuts (especially peanuts)
10. Sesame seeds (similar in make-up to nuts)

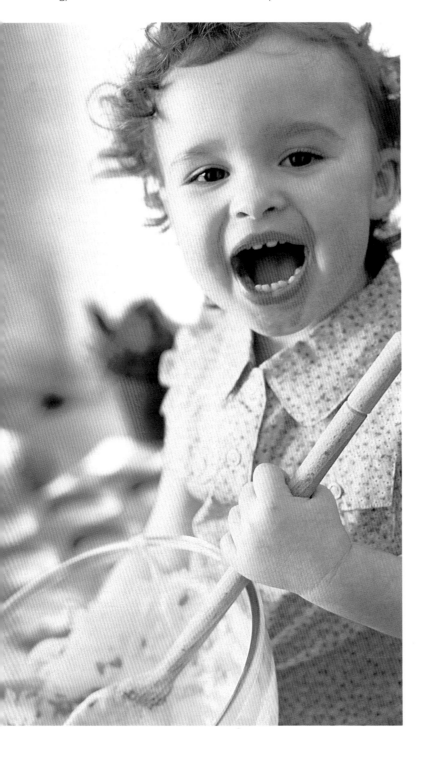

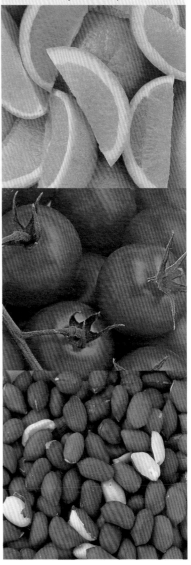

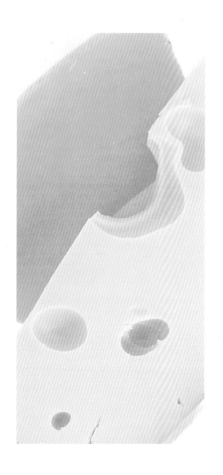

The problem with dairy foods

It might seem incongruous that a child can have a delayed food reaction to cow's milk when he has been quite satisfied with his own mother's breast milk, but the answer lies in the differences in their compounds. Mother's milk contains a much higher content of essential fatty acids than cow's milk, which is one of the reasons for the development of cradle cap when an infant is weaned off the breast.

In addition, all commercial dairy cows are now fed antibiotics on a regular basis, to prevent mastitis and other possible infections that they might pick up in the milking houses or out in the fields; and they are often milked more regularly than is natural, because they are also fed hormones to increase their milk production. Consequently the specific cause of the reaction that your child might experience is difficult to determine, but the symptoms are the same.

If a food doesn't agree with your child, there are alternatives. Goat's milk is much closer in molecular structure to mother's milk than cow's milk is, and formula milks have now been developed that are derived from goat's milk. They contain a higher ratio of essential fatty acids, preventing the development of eczema and other skin rashes. Other alternatives include soya milk and rice milk (both of which are used frequently in Oriental countries) and a milk derived from oats, known as Oatly (see Resources, pages 156–7, for further information).

Runny noses and blocked ears

Dairy products are one of the main offenders in the common problems of runny noses (chronic rhinitis) and blocked ears (otitis media). In chronic states, such afflictions often lead to repeated

Dairy-free alternatives

Dairy product	Dairy-free product
Milk	Soya, oat, rice, coconut or almond milk (the last two are quite sweet, and should not be used all the time, because their fat content is higher than that of the others)
Yoghurt	Soya-based (if no acute allergy to soya has been determined), Yofu (tofu yoghurt); goat's or sheep's yoghurt (if no delayed food reaction to all dairy foods has been established)
Cheese	Vegetarian cheese or soya cheese
Butter	Olivio (derived from olive oil) and Vitaquell; use only olive oil for cooking, because other oils become rancid in the heating process
Cream	Soya cream, or almond cream made from ground almonds and water

doses of antibiotics, which do little to remove the symptoms on a permanent basis, because the cause is a food, and not an infection. If your child suffers from glue ear and has been recommended to have grommets fitted, try putting her on a completely dairy-free diet for at least three weeks to see if the symptoms subside, before putting her through the ordeal of an operation. In many cases the subsidence of symptoms is almost immediate; in other cases there may be further contributory factors. It is an easy test, and one that your child will welcome the opportunity of trying if she suffers regularly from problems with her hearing.

A constantly runny nose is a classic symptom of a delayed food reaction – dairy products being the most common culprit. Apply the same rules of exclusion for at least three weeks to determine whether or not this (or any other frequently consumed food) may be at the root of the problem.

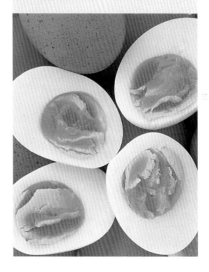

What's getting under your child's skin?

Frequently children develop a number of skin irritations, ranging from dry skin patches to full-blown eczema. In its worst state, eczema can be extremely distressing for a young infant, who will scratch himself until he is bleeding. Acute food allergies have been found to be a major (but not the sole) cause of such problems. It is recommended that you work with a nutrition consultant or other health practitioner to determine the specific foods that may be the cause, and to look at the alternatives to ensure that your child is not missing out on vital nutrients during his growth spurt.

The trouble with wheat

Much has been written about wheat, the ubiquitous grain which should supply your child with an abundance of essential nutrients. However, over the past 20 years or so the refining of wheat has become a commercial art in itself, eliminating as much as 70–80 per cent of its vital nutrients. Wheat flour is now found in virtually every bread, cake, breakfast cereal, biscuit, chocolate treat and pasta, as well as many puddings. There are many recipe books that have been adapted to include recipes for those who may be wheat allergic or gluten-sensitive (coeliac disease). Symptoms of gluten sensitivity may include skin problems, blocked ears or nose, fatigue or extreme drowsiness shortly after eating.

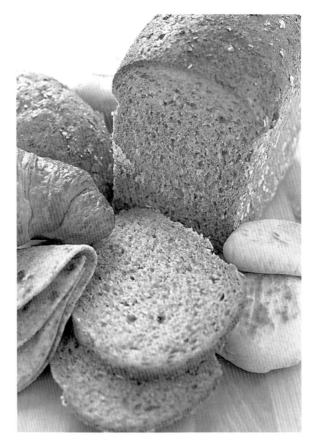

What is gluten sensitivity?

Gluten is the protein portion of four main grains – wheat, oats, rye and barley (although the gluten content in oats is markedly lower than that in the three other grains). It has a tendency to create a glue-like consistency in the digestive tract, which may interfere with your child's nutrient absorption. Gluten sensitivity is known as coeliac disease. If your child suffers from constant diarrhoea, an inability to put on weight and regular stomach pain, you should take him to see a doctor or specialist to determine whether he might have this debilitating condition. Although rare, coeliac disease is now recognized as a genuine childhood illness and early detection is vital as it may determine the health of your child for the rest of his life.

Top tip
Cutting out ALL grains for two to three weeks will give a clear indication of whether or not these foods are causing your child problems with his digestion as symptoms may improve dramatically.

The issue with nuts

Broadly speaking, genuine acute nut allergies are very rare, but today most schools operate a 'nut-free' policy, as this type of acute allergy – known as anaphylaxis (or toxic shock) – can be life-threatening. The extremely high level of histamine released in response to an allergen in nuts can send a child into semi- or total unconciousness within minutes, or even halt their breathing. It is now believed that the acute allergy is to a specific mould found in nuts, particularly that of peanuts.

If there is already someone in your family with an acute nut allergy, it is recommended that you do not eat nuts during pregnancy, and that you are tested for any intolerance level prior to breastfeeding. If one child in the family has a severe nut allergy, then all nuts should be kept out of the house, because even the mould spores in the air can have an effect on a sensitive child.

Wheat alternatives	
Grains	Buckwheat (rhubarb family, and not from the wheat family), rye, oats, millet, corn, barley, rice
Pasta	Corn, buckwheat or barley pasta, and rice noodles
Cereals	Porridge oats, muesli made from millet and barley flakes with oats, corn flakes, rice-puff cereals
Bread	Rye-flour soda breads, pumpernickel, rice cakes, oat cakes, and special gluten-free breads (available by prescription on the NHS for those diagnosed with coeliac disease)
Flours for baking	Rye flour, barley flour, buckwheat flour (for pancakes), soya flour, corn flour, and special wheat-free flours (see Resources, pages 156–7)

The link with sesame

Sesame seeds (unlike sunflower seeds, pumpkin seeds and linseeds) are similar to nuts and should also be avoided by any child with an acute nut allergy. Sesame seeds are often used to flavour Oriental dishes, so take great care to note all the ingredients in any pre-packaged food.

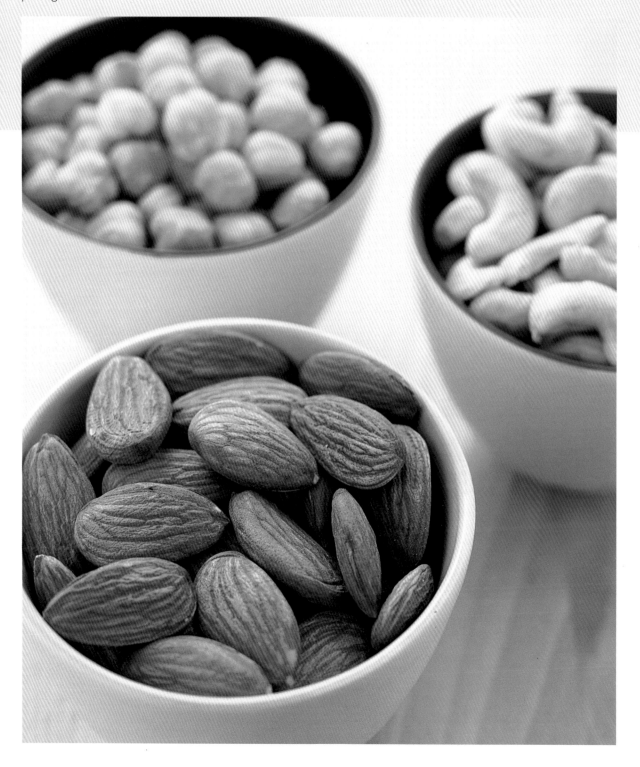

Recognizing hyperactivity

Some children are more chemically sensitive than others to foods, additives and colourings, sugars and sweeteners. If your child exhibits wild behaviour, lack of concentration, violent mood swings or outbursts of temper, kicking, biting and other destructive patterns, he may well be hyperactive. The degree to which these sensitivities exhibit themselves varies hugely, and it is important to understand fully the basis of your own child's problem.

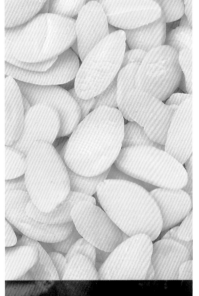

Orthodox treatment offers several recognized drugs that can subdue and calm the most hyperactive of children, but these are chemicals themselves and merely reduce the symptoms of the problem, rather than addressing the root cause. It is advisable to get a proper medical diagnosis in the first instance, together with allergy tests to look at the most common foods and environmental toxins that may be affecting your child.

Feingold's formula

Dr Ben Feingold practised naturopathic principles of medicine (that is, letting the body heal itself when given what it needs). He discovered that most hyperactive children are sensitive to chemicals, colourings and additives, and to a group of naturally occurring chemicals known

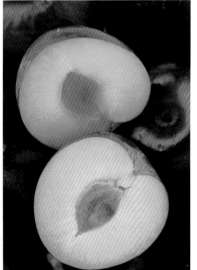

Salicylate-rich foods

It is important to identify which of these foods your child has a craving for, or eats an abundance of, because it is probable that this is the very food that is causing the problem. The two most likely irritants are tomatoes and orange-flavoured drinks and snacks.

Oranges	Tomatoes	Grapes	Plums
Almonds	Cherries	Nectarines	Peppers
Apples	Cranberries	Tangerines	Prunes
Apricots	Cucumbers	Peaches	Raisins

It is interesting to note that this list includes almost all dried fruits (which are also high in sugars), as well as many of the orange-coloured fruits.

as salicylates in seemingly 'healthy' foods. These have aspirin-like qualities that cause reactions in children (and adults) who are particularly sensitive to them. They are found in the foods given in the list on page 70.

The orange of tartrazine

The most abundant orange colouring used in children's food and drink is tartrazine. This chemical was invented in the 1960s to add orange colouring to cola drinks, chocolate fillers and icings on cakes and jellies. It is possibly the most reactive type of food chemical currently on the market, and its safety is currently being questioned in the USA, where the authorities are considering banning tartrazine from all food products.

Check carefully the ingredients of any ready-made food that you give your child – tartrazine and other colourings are often listed way down on the list and can easily be missed. You may suspect any cola, squash or pudding with a bright-orange colouring to contain this chemical.

The role of EFAs

EFAs (essential fatty acids), particularly of the omega-3 group, have been found to be deficient in many children with Attention Deficit Hyperactivity Disorder (otherwise known as ADHD). Essential fats make up a large part of the outer layer of the highly sensitive brain and nerve cells that transmit information and reactions to each other. A lack of these fats may result in incomplete or over-active communication between the cells, leading to the aberrant patterns of behaviour that your child may be exhibiting. EFAs are found mainly in oily fish (such as sardines, salmon and tuna, herrings and mackerel), so it is important to look at the consumption of these foods in your child. If she does not choose fish as a main food, or is vegetarian, it may be necessary to supplement her diet with linseed capsules or oil, which have a higher content of omega-3 essential fats than the other seed oils.

In all cases your child's diet – and sensitivities – may best be worked out with a nutritionist or allergy specialist, who is able to recommend a properly balanced diet, designed to minimize the risk of vitamin deficiencies.

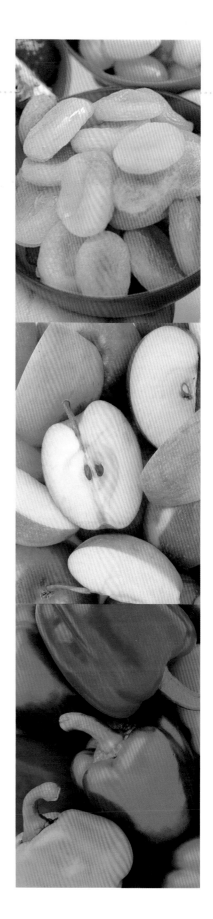

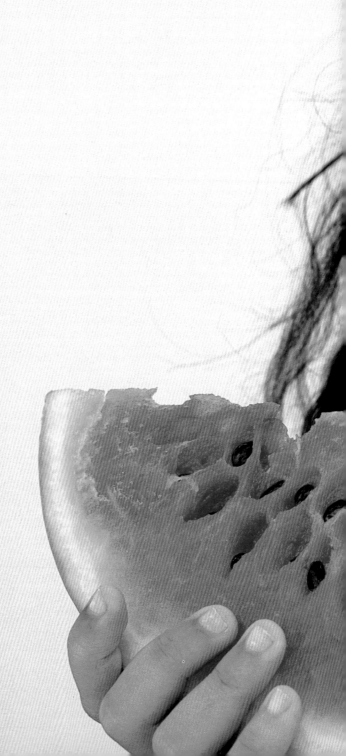

PART 2

Nutrition for growing bodies and minds

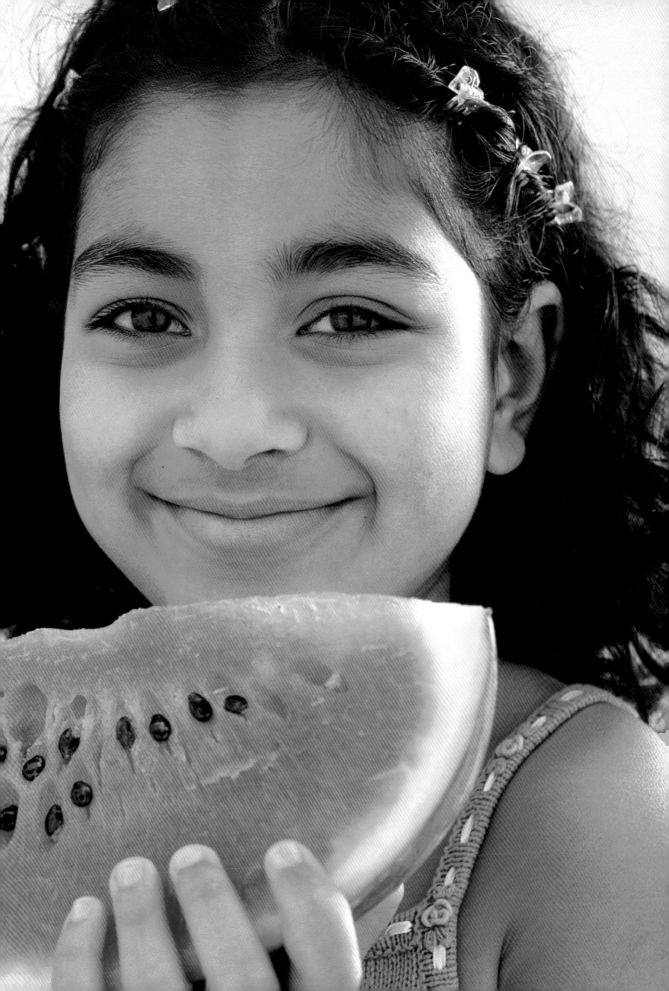

Nutrients for development

B vitamins
Beta-carotene
Calcium
Essential fatty acids
Selenium
Vitamin A
Vitamin K
Zinc

The development of your child in the first six months is a wonder to behold. Feeding and sleeping appear to be your child's only interests initially, but, internally, all the systems of the body are developing at the same amazing pace that occurred prior to birth. Maintaining regular feeds will allow for optimum development of body and brain, as growth and development are encouraged from moment to moment.

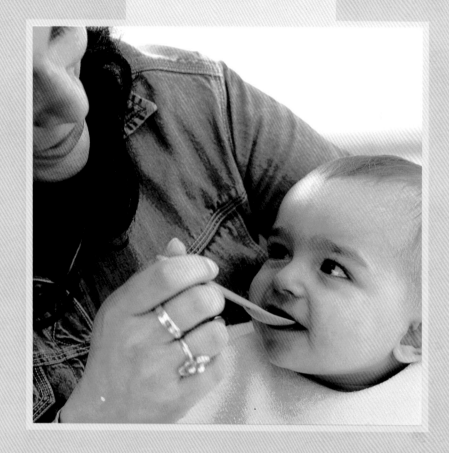

0-6

Birth to six months

Stages of development

The first six months of a child's life exhibit the fastest growth of all, excluding development in the womb, with visible changes taking place almost daily. While breast milk feeds and protects the immune system, the rest of the body is adapting to the outside world, as limbs stretch out to every new stimulus around them.

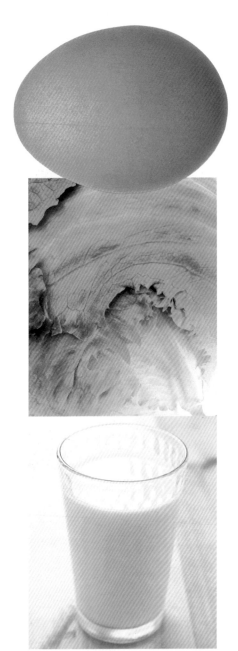

This is a period when maternal instinct shields the child from every observable challenge, although the infant body wriggles its way towards every new experience, as if craving the new information.

Brain food

The first 16 weeks of life are critical for the development of brain tissue. At birth, the brain weighs approximately 25 per cent of its total adult weight. (The ratio of the head to the body at birth is 1:4, reducing to 1:8 by adulthood.) The main nutrients required by the brain at this time are essential fatty acids (found primarily in breast milk, and derived from the mother's consumption of omega-3 fats from fish sources, and omega-6 fats from vegetarian nuts, seed, oils and wholegrains). Where these are lacking in the mother's diet, they are derived from whichever available stores she may have in her body. This is one of the reasons why many women suffer from dry skin and hair loss during the first few months of nursing, because their own fat stores dry out, leaving little for their personal needs.

Essential fatty acids are vital for the development of the brain and nervous system, and whilst it is important to supply these throughout the entire growth of your child, it is particularly crucial at this stage, when the development of the nerve cells is so rapid. It is not enough to supply a child with the outside stimuli of sound, sight and taste – the growth must also come from within. Essential fats are also important for keeping your baby warm, with approximately 25 per cent of his weight being fat, helping to regulate body temperature.

Where breastfeeding is not an option, it is important to ensure that you select the most appropriate type of formula milk for your child (see From Breast to bottle, pages 12–15).

Baby bones

It is well known that calcium is one of the most important minerals for the growth of bone and ligament tissue, particularly in children, and the daily requirement from birth to six months is 400 mg per day, which is primarily provided by breast and formula milk. Movement at this stage is known as 'rhythmic stereotype', in which the body strives to improve simple motor control (reaching for the breast, stretching out the hands – all performed under reflex motor action).

The breath of life

At birth, the breathing airways of the infant are undeveloped and limited, and it is important to ensure that nothing obstructs her breathing, either when awake or asleep. If your child is having trouble breathing, do not hesitate to check with a medical practitioner that nothing is impeding her natural breathing. Or look at what you, as a mother, are consuming, because food sensitivity through the mother's breast milk may be causing inflammation of the airways, or congested mucus (see Allergies and intolerances, pages 64–9). Remember that if the mother is intolerant to certain foods, she may pass on those sensitivities to her infant while breastfeeding. It is important, in this instance, to work with a nutrition consultant or other qualified practitioner to identify potential food culprits.

Gut reaction

At birth, the digestive tract of the newborn is sterile, which is one of the reasons why all babies are given an injection of vitamin K, which is vital for blood clotting. The mother's intake of cabbage and cauliflower helps to increase the natural level of this vitamin that she may already have in her system.

Any reaction a baby may have to a foodstuff at this age is likely to be severe, because beneficial and protective bacteria are only available in small numbers, and the digestive system is immature. It is therefore important for the mother to eat plenty of fresh and raw foods in order to pass on the best possible nutrient variety and content to her baby. Consuming large amounts of coffee, tea and other stimulants is likely to make a baby nervous and restless, as well as causing diarrhoea and colic.

It is not until the age of five to six months that the reflex of sucking and chewing simultaneously occurs, and this is one of the reasons for not weaning onto first foods too quickly. By six months, your baby is capable of swallowing and holding food in the mouth, or spitting it out.

Maximizing immunity

From the moment of birth your baby is exposed to a myriad of bacteria and other potential sources of harm. The immune system is

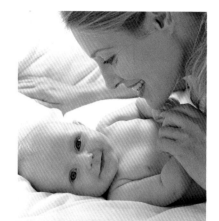
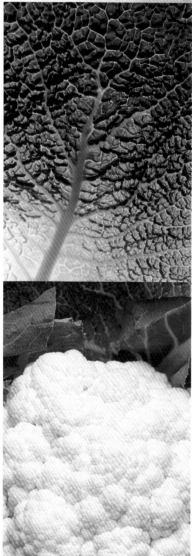

Signs of a lack of essential fats

There are several symptoms that may indicate an insufficiency of essential fats in your baby's diet. They include:

- Poor hair growth
- Dry scalp (cradle cap)
- Cracked skin around the heels and elbows
- Scaly skin on the face and neck
- Eczema-type rash and itchiness anywhere on the body.

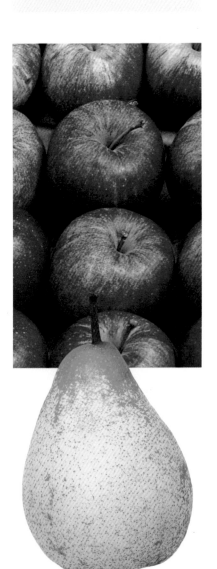

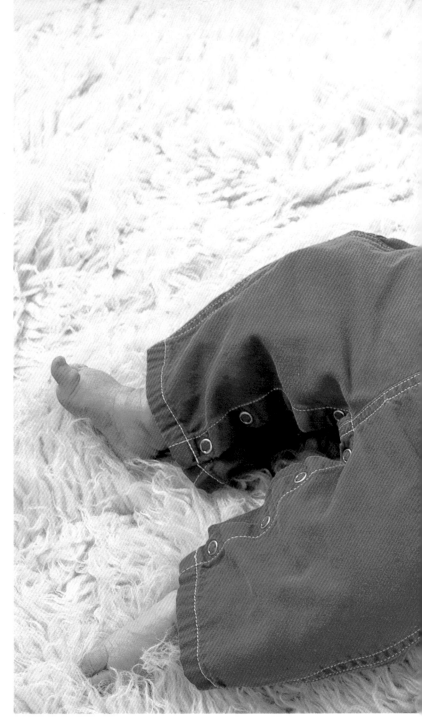

complex and depends on many nutrients to develop. As a large percentage of the immune system is held in the digestive tract, it is important to ensure that everything offered by mouth is properly sterilized during the first few months, to prevent unnecessary infections. Essential nutrients are initially found mainly in the colostrum of the mother's milk (provided during the first three to four days after birth), and subsequently in breast milk and formulas. For this reason it is important to follow the manufacturer's directions when making up formula milk and not to dilute more than is suggested.

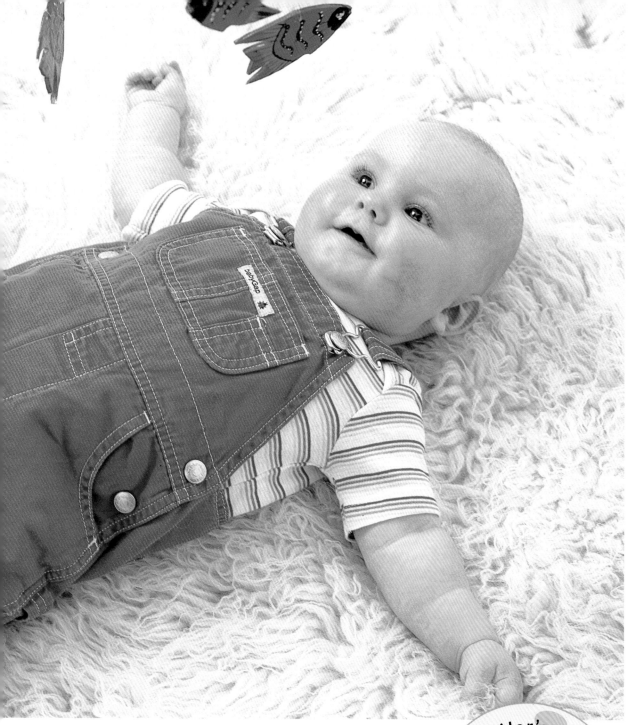

Eye see

It is a common misconception that babies cannot see or focus, or that they only see in black and white. In fact, by the age of three months they can focus on objects and discriminate colours as well as adults can, although they may not recognize what they are looking at.

Vitamin A (retinol) and its precursor, beta-carotene, are essential for good eyesight, and all red, orange and yellow vegetables and fruits are high in these nutrients. The mother's consumption of these foods may go a long way towards enhancing the development of her child's sight.

Toddler's top tip

Keep your child contented and calm with regular feeds that he can rely on. Crying at this stage is usually a sign of hunger or being tired – easy to remedy!

When and why to wean

The speed of growth can vary hugely from one child to another, and it is important to understand for yourself when the time has come to wean your child from just bottle or breast to requiring more than that.

Reasons for weaning

- Restless and interrupted sleep
- Dissatisfaction with breast or bottle
- Mother returning to work
- Milk supply drying up, or proving insufficient
- Maternal unhappiness with the process of breast-feeding
- Excessive sleepiness in a baby.

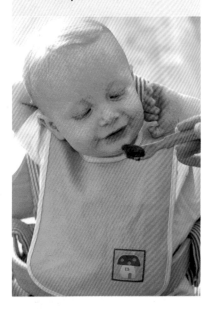

Much is written about when is the optimal time to wean, and this can be confusing to many mothers. As a general guide, babies will show signs of looking for something more than just milk. Use your instincts and your awareness of changes in your child's eating patterns, his demands for feeding, and apparent energy or lethargy. If your child has become restless and seems to be dissatisfied, even after feeding from the breast, he may not be full and it may be time to look at providing first foods.

For a guide as to when to wean your baby, see the following chart of feed frequencies to gauge whether or not your child is getting as much as he needs.

Weaning whys and wherefores

- Pick a time when there are few distractions for both you and your baby.
- Introduce single-grain cereal first. This can be mixed with breast or bottle milk, so that initially it is not much thicker than milk itself, but will 'plop' from the spoon. Start with just one or two teaspoons at a time.
- Always use a spoon for feeding solids, even when offering thinned cereals. Feeding from a bottle not only defeats the object of learning to eat from a spoon, but can also cause choking, as the infant may receive too much food at once.
- Don't be discouraged if your baby at first rejects both spoon and cereal. Try again next time in a relaxed and calm manner.
- Follow cereal with puréed fruits such as apples and pears (good first fruits) and vegetables (see First solid foods, pages 90–91).
- Introduce each food one at a time (not as a blend), every three to four days – this will determine any possible reactions or intolerances.
- Take your time, and don't give up; this is a learning process for both parent and child!

Suggested feeding frequencies

If you are using formula milks, follow the recommended dosage and do not alter this without medical advice, as it has been carefully quantified to offer your child optimum nutritional status.

Cow's milk formula

Age (weeks/months)	Weight (in kg)	(lbs ozs)	No. of feeds per day	Cooled boiled water (in ml)	(lbs ozs)	Level scoops of powder
up to 2 weeks	3.5	7.7	6	85	2.8	3
2–4 weeks	3.9	8.6	5	115	3.8	4
4–8 weeks	4.7	10.3	5	140	4.7	5
8–12 weeks	5.4	11.9	5	170	5.7	6
3–4 months	6.2	13.6	5	170	5.7	6
4–5 months	6.9	15.2	5	200	6.7	7
5–6 months	7.6	16.7	5	200	6.7	7

Goat's milk

Age (months)	Average weight (in kg)	(lbs ozs)	No. of feeds per day	Cooled boiled water (in ml)	(lbs ozs)	Level scoops of powder
0–1	up to 4	8.8	6	90	3	3
1–2	4–5	8.8–11	5	150	5	5
3–5	6–7	13.2–15.4	5	210	7	7

SMA formula milk

Age (weeks/months)	Weight (in kg)	(lbs ozs)	No. of feeds per day	Cooled boiled water (in ml)	(lbs ozs)	Level scoops of powder
Birth	3.5	7.7	6	85	2.8	3
2 weeks	4	8.8	6	115	3.8	4
2 months	5	11	5	170	5.7	6
4 months	6.5	14.3	5	200	6.7	7
6 months	7.5	16.5	4	225	7.6	8

Care when heating baby food

- Take care when heating food in a microwave, which can create pockets of heat that may be too hot for a baby. Stir foods well after heating, and always test the temperature by putting a small amount on your bottom lip – it should feel warm, but not hot.
- Always take baby food out of the jar and put it into a small, shallow container. This will help keep any food that remains in the jar free from bacterial contamination.

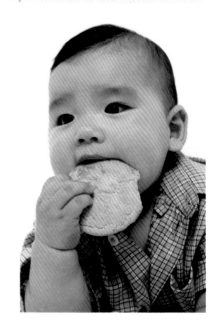

Problems and solutions

The main problems that occur at this age relate to changing needs and changing diet, both of which occur relatively rapidly, as this is one of the fastest growth spurts of a child's life. Responding to your child's needs on a daily basis can be both frustrating and exhausting, because you want to encourage them to regard first foods with interest and joy, but it isn't always that simple.

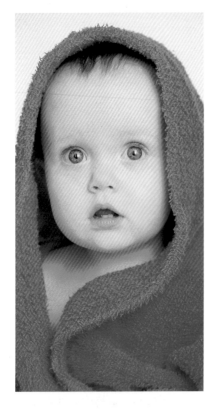

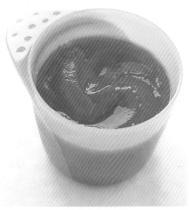

The rate at which your baby grows will inevitably dictate his changing needs, and the wider the variety of foods you can introduce at the weaning and first-foods stage, the better. Some children are much fussier than others, and it may seem impossible at first to entice your child to try new flavours. Remaining calm and interested are the key prerequisites for a relaxed mealtime, and it is recommended that you do not introduce a new food or juice immediately prior to bedtime, as this may upset your baby's sleep pattern.

Food rejection

Specific nutrient deficiencies can become noticeable at an early age, particularly if your baby seems to be underweight, and unhappy at mealtimes. Underweight babies are always carefully monitored to check if there might be a problem with absorption through the digestive tract. It may be that, initially, all foods are rejected. If this happens in a dramatic way (for instance, if your baby suffers from vomiting or develops chronic diarrhoea), you should consider the possibility of a digestive problem and seek medical help.

However, if your baby simply appears to be fussy about trying new foods in the first place, without the physical side-effects mentioned above, take a little more time over introducing foods and let her smell and look at them, prior to expecting her to devour them.

At this age, changing from breast to formula, or from formula to first purées, can elicit noticeable reactions, such as cradle cap, skin irritations, or redness and rashes anywhere on the body. While cradle cap is a symptom of a lack of essential fats in the diet, skin rashes and irritations are more likely to be a sign of a mild to moderate food sensitivity.

Dairy produce is high on the allergenic list, and so care must be taken when weaning. Dairy produce is linked to upper respiratory-tract infections, and to glue ear (otitis media), as well as many skin complaints. Likewise for wheat-based foods (including cereals), as these

Suggested remedies

Problems	Solutions
Cradle cap	Ensure no dairy or citrus fruits have been included in the diet; increase the intake of essential fats by ensuring adequate breast or formula milk is being supplied, and reduce the amount of water-based purées until the problem is rectified.
Dry skin on face or body	This is a classic symptom of lack of essential fats from breast milk or formula; if it occurs only after introducing first foods, make up some of the purées with formula milk (nanny-goat has the highest essential fat content) to ensure sufficient levels of these nutrients.
Rash on bottom, arms or legs	This is a prime indication of a food sensitivity and all new foods should be taken out of the diet and then re-introduced one by one, once the skin has settled; avoid introducing tomatoes too early, as these fruits are very acidic.
Colic/tummy cramps	This may indicate a food sensitivity, or food that is too acidic; some young babies cannot tolerate bananas at too young an age, as they are quite rich for the undeveloped digestive tract. Preparing a weak solution of baby rice water is an excellent antidote to colic. If this problem occurs after introducing a new formula milk, you may wish to try another brand or type, and leave first purées until the problem has been resolved.
Sleeplessness/ restlessness	Some foods are more stimulating and others more sedating. Bananas contain a protein known as tryptophan, which can encourage relaxation and sound sleep in babies who have become restless. Combining a purée with formula or breast milk before bed may help your child to sleep longer, as it will be more satisfying than milk on its own.
Constipation	Any changes in bowel habit or regularity are a primary indication of maladaption to a new food. Infants may pass stools several times per day, but less frequently is not a cause for concern, although constipation needs to be treated early and effectively before it becomes a problem. If your child becomes constipated for no apparent reason, check that she is getting sufficient fluids in her diet. Changing to first foods too quickly, or cutting down on breast/bottle too soon, can both be causes of constipation.
Diarrhoea	This is also a potential hazard, as young babies can become dehydrated very rapidly, which places an enormous burden on their vulnerable kidneys; make sure that your child does not sleep in too hot a room at night, and that fluids are given every two to three hours up to the age of seven to nine months except at night. If you are travelling with a young baby, seek medical advice to prevent such problems occurring. Water with a small amount of a non-citrus juice is ideal for maximizing the absorption of fluids.

are mucus-forming and may irritate a baby's delicate gut lining. Although it is easier, in the short term, to use many of the commercially produced baby products, including pasta, it is best to avoid these for at least the first 12 months to reduce the likelihood of your baby developing intolerant reactions to such foods.

Meal planners

Having looked at the weaning process, it is useful to know which first foods should be introduced at this age. To prevent the possibility of food intolerances, certain foods should not be given to your child at the outset.

Ideal starter foods

There are a number of foods that are most suitable for introducing first. They include:

- Apple
- Pear
- Papaya
- Banana
- Avocado
- Broccoli
- Carrot
- Potato
- Sweet potato
- Squash or pumpkin
- Baby or brown rice

All these fruits and vegetables are suitable for cooking and puréeing to a fine texture. This is important, because a baby can easily choke on anything more bulky or lumpy at this stage. They also include the sweetest of the vegetables, offering plenty of carbohydrate for energy and vitamins for immune development and protection.

Back to basics

Ensure that all fruits and vegetables are fresh, and that they have had their skins removed to reduce the level of pesticides and other chemicals that may be lurking there. Wherever possible, select organic produce for this reason. Only cook as much as you need for one or two feeds. It is not advisable to cook in large quantities for freezing into food cubes until you know that your baby likes a particular food.

Selecting mainly vegetables, and some fruits with baby rice, is the ideal starting point. See the recipe section on First foods (pages 130–33) for ideas and cooking times, and experiment with your own combinations. Minimal kitchen equipment, such as a food processor, will make your work much faster and simpler, and will allow you to try foods on your baby that would otherwise be difficult to purée finely enough. It is important to ensure that all utensils and dishes are sterilized properly, to reduce the possibility of bacterial infection; it is not advisable to use old or recycled utensils at this stage.

Milk

If you are breastfeeding, you may wish to feed on demand, which will allow your child to feed up to eight or nine times per day. It is recommended that you offer your child both breasts at each feed, rather than favouring one or the other breast. This ensures that your baby gets the full nutritional content of the milk – most of the essential fats in human breast milk (which are needed for the development of the nervous system, brain cells and skin) tend to come through at the beginning of each feed, so offering both breasts increases their intake.

If you are using formula milks, follow the recommended dosage and do not alter this without medical advice, as it has been carefully quantified to offer your child optimum nutritional status (see When and why to wean, pages 80–81). If your baby appears to be suffering from colic or reflux, or even projectile vomiting, it may be that the formula you have selected is not the most suitable one. Seek the advice of a nutritionist or other health-care practitioner prior to changing formulas.

Weekly chart for first foods and purées

First foods can be introduced at any time from four months onwards, but larger babies may need some fruit purées one or two weeks earlier. See First foods (pages 130–33) for recipe ideas and methods for preparing first purées.

WEEK 1

6–7 a.m.	Breast/bottle
9–10 a.m.	Breast/bottle
1.30–2 p.m.	Breast/bottle
3–4.30 p.m.	Water or diluted apple juice: 150 ml (5 fl oz)
5.30–6.30 p.m.	Breast/bottle

WEEK 2

6–7 a.m.	Breast/bottle
9–10 a.m.	Breast/bottle and 1–2 teaspoons apple purée
1.30–2 p.m.	Breast/bottle
3–4.30 p.m.	Water or diluted apple or pear juice: 150 ml (5 fl oz)
5.30–6.30 p.m.	Breast/bottle and 3 teaspoons rice

WEEK 3

6–7 a.m.	Breast/bottle
9–10 a.m.	Breast/bottle and 3–4 teaspoons apple or pear purée
1.30–2 p.m.	Breast/bottle and 1–2 teaspoons root-vegetable purée
3–4.30 p.m.	Water or fruit juice
5.30–6.30 p.m.	Bottle, 4 teaspoons rice and 2 teaspoons fruit purée

WEEK 4

6–7 a.m.	Breast/bottle
9–10 a.m.	Breast/bottle and 5–7 teaspoons fruit purée
1.30–2 p.m.	Breast/bottle and 3–5 teaspoons root-vegetable purée
3–4.30 p.m.	Water or fruit juice and 2 teaspoons banana purée
5.30–6.30 p.m.	Bottle, 4 teaspoons rice and 4 teaspoons fruit purée

From Week 5 you may offer as much of the fruit and vegetable purées as your baby demands, as she will now have a taste for more. Do not force new flavours on her without first allowing her to smell it (remember that digestion begins with sight and smell). You may want to increase the number of feeds now to six times daily, including the bedtime bottle or breast feed, as her appetite increases, and you want to encourage sleeping through the night to become part of the routine.

WEEK 5

6–7 a.m.	Fruit purée with rice
9–10 a.m.	Breast/bottle
1.30–2 p.m.	Mixed root-vegetable purée
3–4.30 p.m.	Breast/bottle
5.30–6.30 p.m.	Mixed fruit purée
Bedtime	Breast/bottle

WEEK 6

6–7 a.m.	Mixed fruit purée
9–10 a.m.	Breast/bottle and banana purée
1.30–2 p.m.	Potato and green vegetable purée
3–4.30 p.m.	Breast/bottle
5.30–6.30 p.m.	Mixed vegetable purée
Bedtime	Breast/bottle

This should just about take you to the six-month-plus age group, which is covered in the next section (if it doesn't, simply repeat Weeks 5 and 6 as necessary, introducing new fruits or vegetables every five to six days to monitor for any possible intolerant reactions). If your baby has taken first foods at a later age, do not rush into the next phase before going through these early weaning fruits and vegetables, as they are the most suitable foods to introduce, as well as breast or formula milk.

Nutrients for development

B-complex vitamins
(specifically B1, B3 and B6)
Boron
Calcium
Essential fats
Magnesium
Manganese
Vitamin C
Vitamin D

Your baby is now becoming an active person, and his sight, touch, smell and taste are becoming more developed. It is during this stage that first foods are introduced, and a wider variety of nutrients are needed to encourage healthy development of the skeletal system, which in turn allows sitting, crawling, standing and walking. Giving your child new foods also increases his digestive capabilities.

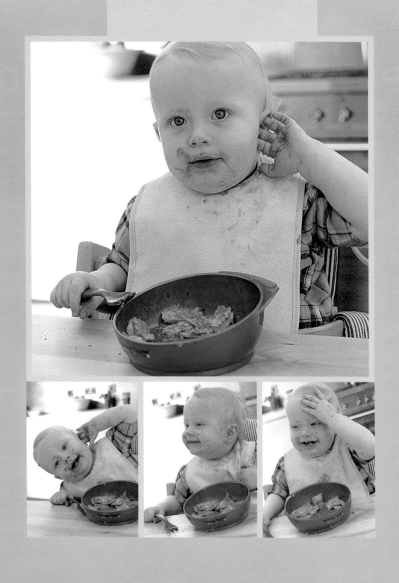

2-18

Seven to eighteen months

Stages of development

During the first two years the body grows more rapidly than at any time after birth. This age group shows the greatest development of nervous and cognitive functions – that is, the brain, sight, hearing and smell, as well as physical coordination and speech. Most of the brain cells in the part of the brain known as the cerebrum, which govern these controls, are fully developed by 18 months, although the parts that control movement and posture (the cerebellum and brain stem) are only about 60 per cent developed by the time the child has mastered the balance required to stand and walk.

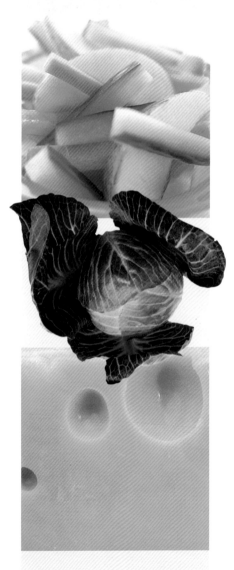

Walkie-talkie

This is an important time for muscle and skeletal development, as the infant transgresses from propping himself up to crawling, and eventually to standing and walking. At eight months, children have the muscle strength to sit up, and the lumbar curve appears. It is therefore important to ensure that the range of foods increases substantially at this age to allow for such rapid development.

Teeth also grow rapidly at this stage, requiring the same nutrients for development as bone. Poor teeth growth is an indication of problems with digestion or absorption, or of a child who is not being given sufficient solid foods to 'cut his teeth on' – literally.

It is also during this period that a child's ability to see reaches that of an adult, with depth of field, colour and minor details all being within their grasp. This partly explains why children of this age are so inquisitive and constantly point to objects, saying 'See' or naming specific people and things.

Protein power

The appetite of a child growing at this rate changes dramatically, with demands for new tastes, textures and flavours being an important part of the learning process. Progressing from simple purées and milk to first solid foods and actual meals is a vital stage, with the demand for a wider range of protein foods increasing, as growth is dependent on it.

Remember that proteins are the building blocks of your child's body, and a selection of animal- and vegetable-based proteins should be included increasingly in every meal at this stage. Chicken, fish and some meats may be introduced gradually throughout this age group, as your child's appetite becomes larger. Pulses, chickpeas, lentils and beans of all kinds are valuable sources of protein, not only for the

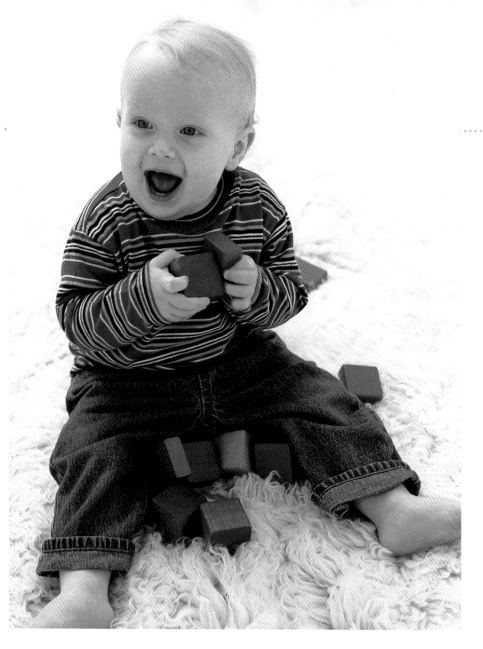

vegetarian child, but for those who choose to eat animal protein too. Beans and pulses are an excellent source of calcium to replace milk and dairy products, which may not be tolerable to some young babies (with lactose intolerance). So too are green leafy vegetables (particularly those that 'stand tall', such as broccoli, celery and cauliflower), with the added bonus of also containing magnesium, which is vital for calcium absorption.

Vitamin vitality

Collagen is required for the formation of bone, and not just for healthy plump young skin! The most important nutrient to support collagen formation is vitamin C, which must be consumed daily, as it cannot be stored in the body. Including potatoes, green peppers, cabbage, melon, broccoli and sweet potatoes (as well as all the citrus fruits and tomatoes) will provide a good variety of foods that are all rich in vitamin C. Vitamin C and D are also essential for the absorption of calcium into bone, so these nutrients all work in harmony.

Watching your child playing as well as eating will give you an indication of what might be missing. Many children of this age will pick up earth, stones and other mineral-loaded items from the garden and surroundings – this is a sign that their iron status may be below par. See the chart of vitamins and minerals on pages 152–5 to identify the different nutrients required, and those foods that are richest in them.

First solid foods

Children at this age become increasingly inquisitive about the food around them – they notice everything their parents are eating, and frequently stretch out to reach foods that are aimed for parental mouths. At this point you should start giving them their first solid foods to hold and smell, because all their senses are being stimulated on a moment-to-moment basis.

Finger foods

Vegetables
- Carrots (cut into sticks/batons)
- Celery (strings removed, and cut into quarters, lengthways)
- Swede (cut into strips about 6–8 cm/2½–3 in long)
- Parsnips (as swede)
- Cauliflower (cut lengthways along the stem)
- Sweet potato (cut into batons, as for carrots)
- Red and yellow peppers (cut into strips lengthways, pips removed)

Fruits
- Apples (cut into long strips)
- Unripe pears (cut into strips)
- Pineapple (but not before 10 months)

Toothless wonder

As the milk teeth start to come to the surface of the gums, your baby will instinctively want to press hard objects between his gums to identify this new sensation. It is perfectly normal at this stage for babies to suck and even chew on their own fingers and thumbs, and this should not always be assumed to be a sign of hunger. It is more likely to be an investigative response: how hard can he press his jaws together before he stops? If you offer your own finger to his mouth, you will find that the pressure he applies before stopping is enormously strong!

Babies will put anything in their mouths as they seek to establish the difference between one texture and another. Toys, fingers, hard objects such as pens, pencils and keys – they don't know how to differentiate between them, so it is important to watch them constantly, for it only takes a couple of seconds to pick up an object and it will go straight into the mouth.

Thumb-sucking is a different reflex: as young babies are weaned, they seek a substitute for their mother's breast, and their own fingers and thumbs are the most easily accessible object. The suckling reflex continues long after the weaning process – often for several years – and it is debatable whether or not this should be discouraged at any age, or allowed to subside at your child's own pace.

Bigger bones

Remember that tooth development runs alongside bone development, with the same nutrients required for both. Looking for more solid foods is an indication that the nutrients your child needs are different from what they were a few months ago, when the primary development was brain and nerve tissue. It is also a sign that the chewing reflex is coming into play and, while this is a learned reflex, it pays to stimulate the senses with a selection of different textures.

Raw foods provide the most satisfactory stimulus, as the texture is so different from the purées and mashes offered up to this point. Root vegetables, such as carrots, parsnip and swede, are all appealing for their natural sweetness (but celery can be troublesome during the younger months, as the strings may come away from the stem and get stuck in a baby's throat). Red and green peppers offer a more hydrated and sweet version of root vegetables, as well as being packed with vitamin C, which is needed for bone and teeth development. Fruits such as apples and hard pears are ideal first fruits to introduce in their raw state, and chunks should be offered at the end of a cooked meal to encourage the differentiation between textures.

Lightly cooked, steamed vegetables in bite-sized pieces should also be given so that your baby is encouraged to chew, rather than suck, and learn how much she can or cannot hold in her mouth. You may find, in the beginning, that she cannot gauge how much this is, and does not know how and when to swallow to coordinate the emptying of one mouthful before beginning the next.

Digestive changes

As the choice of foods changes, so does the digestive capability of your child. Whereas it was previously important to provide a range of fruits, vegetables and wholegrains that contained readily available sugars for energy and rapid growth, now the preference is for foods that provide more dense sources of minerals, particularly those needed for bone and teeth development. These include calcium, magnesium, boron, manganese and phosphorus. The majority of these nutrients are found in dairy produce, green leafy and structured vegetables (such as broccoli and celery) and oily fish (such as sardines, tuna and salmon).

Your baby will be less sensitive to new foods now, but that is no excuse to ignore the telltale signs of a possible food intolerance. Diarrhoea, constipation, vomiting, rashes and shortness of breath all indicate an intolerance or even an allergy, and should be noted carefully. At this stage your child may be quite vocal about foods that he likes or dislikes. This does not necessarily indicate a fussy eater: he is just being intuitive about the foods he needs and wants.

Gut flora are more developed now, as are the digestive enzymes, allowing your baby to fully digest and absorb a wider range of foods. Nonetheless, she may veer towards one group of foods more than another, which is perfectly normal.

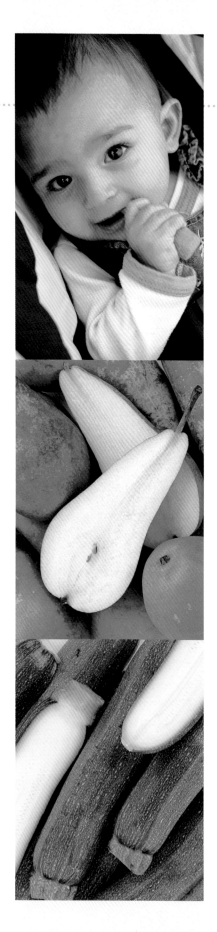

Problems and solutions

Some children develop later than others, but when your child chooses to start eating solid foods may be an indication of rapid development. If his teeth begin to come through early, then he will probably have equally advanced development of the bones in his legs and arms, and may have sat up by himself from an early age.

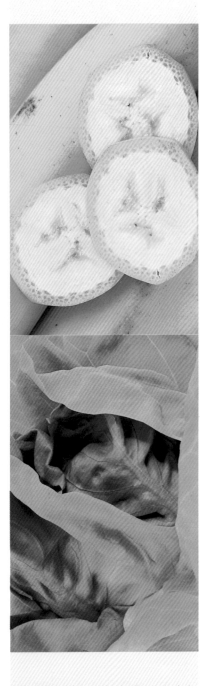

Hand–eye contact

Other indicators of the speed of your child's development include the success with which he can or cannot seem to coordinate crawling and walking, and the movement between hand and mouth when he starts to feed himself. Remember that hand–eye coordination depends on the relevant information in the brain instructing the hand to move towards the mouth accurately – and that an insufficient amount of good-quality essential fats in the diet, coupled with a low intake of B vitamins, may slow the development of the brain cells that instruct movement and coordination.

It is vital that your child is stimulated to develop all these skills. They don't just happen, without the involvement of others to show them how to use their limbs, begin to crawl and subsequently walk. New toys and playthings (as well as spoons and forks at the table) are essential to encourage the development of hand–eye coordination. While your child may initially make a mess of the kitchen, it is only by repetitive trial and error that he will master his own movement!

I can see, I can hear

This is also an important time to notice any difficulties that your child might have with sight, hearing or speech. Some children start uttering words way before others do, and first children are usually slower than their siblings, as parents do not have the experience to know how best to stimulate the development of this function, and the child has no brother or sister to emulate.

If you think your child may be having trouble with sight, hearing or speech, it is always best to seek the advice of a medical practitioner to determine whether or not there is a developmental problem. In the meantime, look at the suggested remedies (see right) to check that you are giving your child all the nutrients he needs to develop those parts of the brain associated with cognitive, auditory and visual function. A narrow or limited diet may be inhibiting the development of one of these vital functions.

Suggested remedies

Problems	Solutions
Poor hand–mouth coordination	Some research indicates beneficial effects of increasing the intake of B vitamins found in barley, rice, buckwheat, corn and millet, bananas and chickpeas. Include plenty of oily fish (tuna, salmon, herring and sardines), as well as sunflower and pumpkin seeds (ground and added to cereals and porridge) to increase the essential fats required for good cognitive function.
Weak or 'lazy bones'	Calcium and magnesium are both essential for the development of strong bones: find them in structured green vegetables (broccoli, cauliflower, cabbage, celery) and all dark-green leaves. The richest sources of calcium are oily fish with small bones (such as salmon and sardines, which can be puréed in the earlier months), all dairy produce (goat's and ewe's dairy, as well as cow's) and all nuts and seeds; almonds may be ground up, and water added, to make a delicious sweet almond milk or cream for younger infants.
Slow teeth growth	As well as calcium, both vitamin C and D are the most important nutrients for the production of collagen, which makes up bones and teeth, so include potatoes, red berry fruits, citrus fruits and their juices, chicken and red meat.
Poor eyesight	Vitamin A and its precursor, beta-carotene, are vital for good eyesight, so include plenty of red, orange and yellow fruits and vegetables (tomatoes, mangoes, apricots, carrots, squash, pumpkin, and red and yellow peppers) in soups and main dishes. Vitamin C is also important (see above on collagen production).
Difficulty in hearing	Excess mucus can preclude your child from hearing properly, and this is most easily recognizable through an inability to imitate or replicate words clearly, or by your child apparently 'ignoring' you when you speak. Excess mucus is a symptom of a dairy intolerance or allergy (see Allergies and intolerances, pages 64–9); foods that help to clear this include those with a high soluble fibre content, such as oats, buckwheat and wholegrain brown rice.

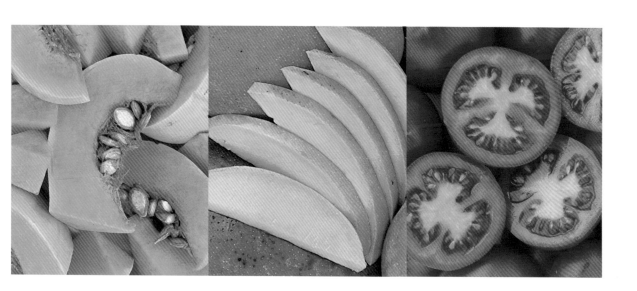

Meal planners

At this stage your child will be starting to hold pieces of food in her own hands and put things in her mouth, to experience the sensation of more solid items.

One-week chart 6 to 12 months

DAY 1

Breakfast	Breast or formula milk with brown rice and peach purée
Mid-morning	Breast or formula milk
Lunch	White-fish, carrot and red-pepper purée
Mid-afternoon	Breast or formula milk
Supper	Avocado and pear purée
Bedtime	Breast or formula milk

DAY 2

Breakfast	Breast or formula milk with quinoa and plum purée
Mid-morning	Breast or formula milk
Lunch	Sweet-potato and red-pepper purée with chicken
Mid-afternoon	Breast or formula milk
Supper	Millet, pear and broccoli purée
Bedtime	Breast or formula milk

DAY 3

Breakfast	Breast or formula milk with oat and apricot purée
Mid-morning	Breast or formula milk
Lunch	Pumpkin, leek and cod purée
Mid-afternoon	Breast or formula milk
Supper	Lentil, red-pepper and tomato purée
Bedtime	Breast or formula milk

DAY 4

Breakfast	Breast or formula milk with brown rice and banana purée
Mid-morning	Breast or formula milk
Lunch	Turkey, potato and pea purée
Mid-afternoon	Breast or formula milk
Supper	Cauliflower, parsnip and butter-nut-squash purée
Bedtime	Breast or formula milk

DAY 5

Breakfast	Breast or formula milk with quinoa and apricot purée
Mid-morning	Breast or formula milk
Lunch	Salmon, potato and sweetcorn purée
Mid-afternoon	Breast or formula milk
Supper	Sweet-potato, carrot and millet purée
Bedtime	Breast or formula milk

DAY 6

Breakfast	Breast or formula milk with oat and papaya purée
Mid-morning	Breast or formula milk
Lunch	Chickpea, tomato and courgette purée
Mid-afternoon	Breast or formula milk
Supper	Potato, pea and spinach purée
Bedtime	Breast or formula milk

DAY 7

Breakfast	Breast or formula milk with brown rice and apple purée
Mid-morning	Breast or formula milk
Lunch	Tuna, butternut-squash and leek purée
Mid-afternoon	Breast or formula milk
Supper	Split-pea and red-pepper purée
Bedtime	Breast or formula milk

One-week chart 12 to 18 months

DAY 1

Breakfast	Oaty porridge with chopped, peeled plums
Lunch	Cod with peas and potato mash
Supper	Well-mashed lentils with tomato and broccoli

DAY 2

Breakfast	Buckwheat porridge and stewed apricots
Lunch	Chopped chicken with puréed sweetcorn and mashed sweet potato
Supper	Root-vegetable mash with carrots, sweet potato and brown rice

DAY 3

Breakfast	Scrambled egg and rye-toast fingers
Lunch	Corn-pasta shapes with steamed and chopped courgettes and broccoli
Supper	Brown-rice risotto with leeks and spinach

DAY 4

Breakfast	Corn-based cereal with bananas and apricots
Lunch	Shepherd's pie with carrots and potatoes
Supper	Orzo with creamy mushroom salsa

DAY 5

Breakfast	Boiled egg (chopped in a cup or bowl) with rye-toast fingers
Lunch	Chicken casserole with pumpkin and tomato mash
Supper	Tagliatelle with a light Cheddar sauce and peas

DAY 6

Breakfast	Oaty porridge with chopped apple and raisins
Lunch	Tuna and red-pepper risotto (made with brown rice)
Supper	Beany balls with diced carrots and sweetcorn purée

DAY 7

Breakfast	Yoghurt and papaya/mango smoothie on rice cereal
Lunch	Beef (or kidney bean) and parsnip casserole with rice and peas
Supper	Baked potato with baked beans and grated cheese

Meal planning: 6–12 months

In the early months of this stage, your baby is still eating puréed foods, but you can introduce new flavours and textures, as well as the animal proteins found in chicken, fish and lean red meats. Green vegetables are important on a daily basis to provide the range of B vitamins, calcium and magnesium required for building strong bones and encouraging teeth formation. You should be feeding your baby six times per day now, with an ongoing combination of breast or formula milk three times daily to ensure optimum nutrient intake.

Meal planning: 12–18 months

Maintain six feeds per day, but start to substitute some of the purées with chopped and mashed fruits, vegetables, chicken and fish, to increase the texture of meals. Also offer more peeled fruits and lightly steamed vegetables for your baby to nibble on. The aim is to encourage him to start chewing by necessity. While he may over-fill his mouth in the early stages, he will soon learn how to chew and swallow before putting in the next mouthful. Maintain mid-morning, mid-afternoon and bedtime (if required) fresh milk feeds according to age, having now weaned from the breast.

Nutrients for development

B-complex vitamins
Essential fatty acids
Omega-3
Omega-6
Vitamin B6
Vitamin C
Zinc

Your child is now eating a much wider variety of foods, and hopefully potty training and a nappy-free existence can be enjoyed. Emotionally your child is already developing his own unique character – talking becomes persistent as he learns new words at a fantastic rate, and moving rapidly on two legs requires constant watching by alert parents!

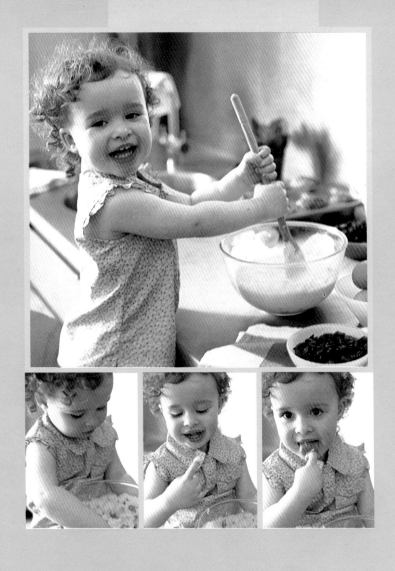

18-3

18 months to 3 years

Stages of development

It is during this age group that digestive function expands, and bladder control is reached (usually around the age of two years).

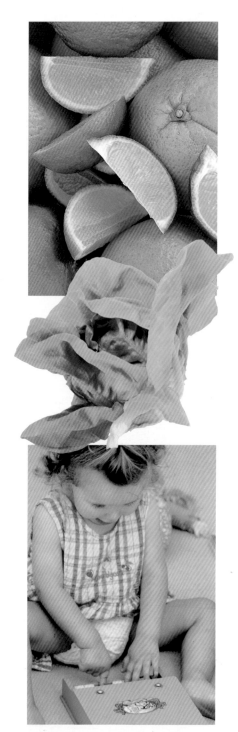

Tummies and bellies

Digestive enzymes, which begin in the mouth and continue in the stomach and small intestine, all develop rapidly at this stage and are essential for the digestion and absorption of a much wider range of foods. At this age children often seek new flavours and textures on an almost weekly basis.

It is vital that the B group of vitamins (found in wholegrains such as brown rice, barley, buckwheat, oats, millet and corn, as well as chicken and turkey, red meat and green leafy vegetables) is supplied in the diet, as the digestive system works around the clock and uses up considerable energy. Broadening the diet is an obvious strategy to ensure a good supply of these essential nutrients.

A weak or poorly developed digestion will show itself in frequent bouts of diarrhoea and weight loss, as well as apparent sensitivity to many of the new foods that are introduced. If you suspect that your child may have a physical problem, it is important to take him to a doctor or specialist to determine which part of the digestive tract is not functioning optimally. Poor digestion leads to the low absorption of essential nutrients for growth and development, poor concentration and constant fatigue. More important conditions such as coeliac disease (see page 68) are rare, but should not be ruled out if your child is losing weight rapidly and seems unable to keep anything down for more than an hour.

Bladder control

Potty training occurs at this stage, requiring both patience and observation, but do not push your child into it if she is reluctant. Some children are much slower than others and there are no set rules, although there are recommendations. It is important to let your child know that this is a natural bodily function and not one that needs to be done behind closed doors, although you may find that she seeks privacy from an early age, emulating your own behaviour.

Bedwetting is likely to occur during the first stages of nappy removal. Never make your child feel ashamed about this natural phenomenon – it is bound to take some time to learn at a subconscious level when he needs to wake to empty his bladder. Bedwetting can cause a lot of anxiety for young children, and there may be a nutritional component to the problem. See if there is the possibility of a mild intolerance to something your child is eating on a regular basis. Citrus fruits and their juices and tomatoes are common culprits, because they are acidic and can irritate the bladder; so too can excess added or refined sugars.

Spine and limbs

By the age of three, movement has become much more refined, as the nervous system is more developed in its coordination and speed of reaction. It is important to provide your child with all the nutrients for the proper development of the spine and brain, which house the core of the nervous system, to allow for speed and agility of movement, as well as sharp mental focus. This is one of the most rapid growth periods for the spinal column (other than when the baby is still in the womb), as the muscular system around it develops to support the full range of flexibility. Essential fatty acids (found in nuts, seeds and their oils, as well as oily fish) are important now for the development of nerve cells in the spine and brain. As your child becomes more active and dextrous with her limbs, so her nutrient intake needs to increase to support this.

The terrible twos

We often wonder what is meant by this phrase until our own children hit it themselves, and then there is no doubt – our beautiful little angels turn into monsters whom we often don't recognize, let alone know how to control. This may be a problem related to changes in blood-sugar levels, nutrient requirements and the growth of metabolic function, as increased energy requirements affect the speed at which food is used up, leaving children irritable and sometimes apparently irrational. As adults, we are prone to reach for a quick-fix stimulant, such as a coffee or some chocolate, but these foods are not appropriate for children of this age, who are much more sensitive to foods and drinks.

To understand more about blood-sugar management, turn to Sugar and spice (pages 38–41),

and look at the glycaemic index of different types of foods. Remember that the higher the score on the glycaemic index, the more rapidly that food will be absorbed and converted into glucose, and hence energy. The more refined the food is, the higher its glycaemic index will be and the more likely your child is to suffer from mood swings. This is particularly obvious if your child has developed a taste for simple sugars, such as those found in squashes, juices and sweet treats.

It is also important to be aware of the possibility of intolerances to certain foods, even totally natural ones. Look at Allergies and intolerances (pages 64–9) and Recognizing hyperactivity (pages 70–71).

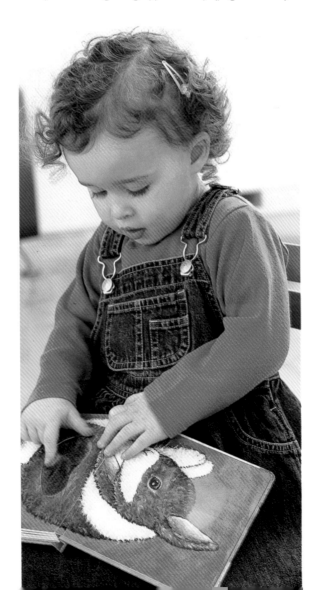

Bigger meals

As your child's rate of growth and energy use increases noticeably, so does the need for larger meals and greater frequency. Ideally your child should go no more than three hours without eating a meal or healthy snack, and it is important to have a ready supply of suitable foods wherever you may be. If you notice that your child has become quiet or lacking in concentration, she may be suffering from low blood-sugar levels, which can be revived within minutes by giving her something to eat.

Good sources of protein

- Milk
- Cheese
- Eggs
- Yoghurt
- Meat
- Fish
- Chicken
- Lentils and other pulses
- Quinoa
- Millet and oat grains
- Nuts (except peanuts) and seeds
- Soya produce (including soya milk and tofu)

Smaller amounts of protein may be derived from vegetables.

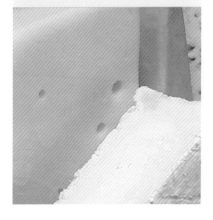

Ups and downs

Some children more than others exhibit the highs and lows in their blood-sugar status. As all food may be converted into glucose at different rates (see Sugar and spice, pages 38–41), it is important to ensure a regular supply of nutrients to the brain and muscles for cognitive function and physical energy. If your child tends to run around with boundless energy for a while, then slumps down exhausted suddenly, his blood-sugar levels may just have taken a nosedive! Up to 70 per cent of all foods digested at this age are used for brain fuel, so keeping your child topped up will enable him to learn and store new information more easily and efficiently. If he is struggling to understand something you are showing him, consider when he ate his last meal.

Main meals

Larger meals will now need to be prepared. Whereas previously you may have served a single dish such as a purée, followed by a pudding, you now need to start preparing several different foodstuffs for the main dish, to avoid your child filling herself up with bread or potatoes. Look to provide some grain or other starch-based carbohydrate with at least two main meals per day (for instance, oats or corn for breakfast, wholegrain bread or pasta for lunch, and rice for tea), and add a source of protein and at least one fruit or vegetable (preferably of different colours) to create an attractive and varied menu. See Meal planners (pages 104–5) for suitable combinations.

As your child goes through growth spurts, she will appear to consume almost disproportionate amounts of food for her size – this is perfectly normal and should not be discouraged.

The protein/carb balance

By including some protein (either from an animal or vegetable source) with every meal or snack, you will prolong the release of energy and ensure a more even temperament in your child. Children will naturally opt for (and sometimes crave) carbohydrates more readily than protein, as their bodies instinctively recognize that they can convert carbohydrates into energy more rapidly than protein. Hence the scenario of a child working his way through all the chips on his plate before even touching the hamburger or fishcake. Allowing him to do this is okay, provided he also eats the protein, as it is in the digestion of both that the correct balance occurs. Eating the carbohydrates on their own will provide a surge of liveliness, followed by apparent fatigue.

Feeding fibre

In an age when many foods have been over-processed, we tend to forget the importance of fibre, and it plays a part in balancing blood-sugar levels for your child. In the digestion and absorption process, fibre slows down the surge of blood sugar and ensures that your child does not become constipated. Make sure that skin is left on apples and other fruits, as this creates a more total food. And grain-based foods should be served in their wholegrain form. Children enjoy muesli and oat or millet porridge for breakfast, and these may all be soaked overnight to reduce preparation time in the morning (see First cereals and breakfast must-haves, pages 134–6).

If you are in the habit of providing your child with fresh fruit juices, remember that all the fibre has been removed in the extraction process, so give a piece of fruit at the same time, to replace some of the natural fibre.

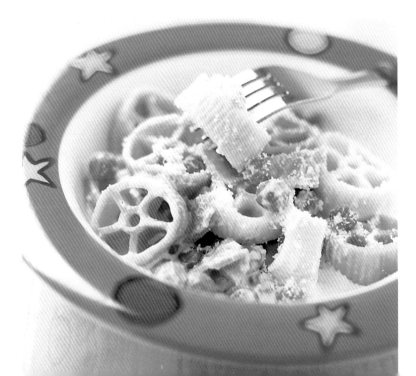

Good sources of carbohydrate

- Cereals
- Biscuits
- Beans and other pulses
- Rice, polenta and other grains
- Pasta
- Polenta pizzas (see page 151)
- All fruits and vegetables
- Wholegrain muffins
- Granola bars

The wholegrain version of any carbohydrate has a higher nutrient content, thereby giving your child more energy for a longer period.

Good sources of natural fibre

- Unpeeled fruits
- Raw vegetables (such as carrots, celery, baby sweet-corn, French beans, mangetout)
- Wholegrain breads
- Oat and rice cakes
- Brown rice
- Wholewheat pasta
- Jacket potatoes (with their skins)
- Baked beans (low-sugar varieties)
- Kidney beans and chickpeas
- Lentils and other pulses

Problems and solutions

There are two main potential problem areas to be dealt with at this stage: one physical and the other mental, since the growth of both body and brain is so rapid. Understanding the extent of a child's nutritional needs has already been explored (see Bigger meals, pages 100–101).

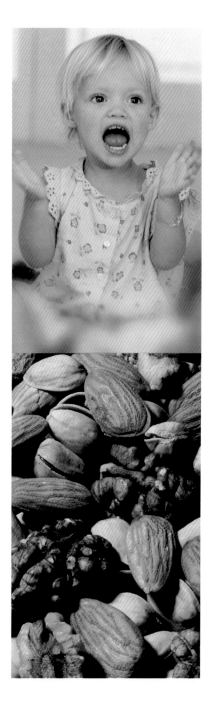

Physical problems

Increasing bone and muscle development requires increased protein at this age, when walking, running and physical activities become much more commonplace. The developing nervous system is important for both physical and mental acuity, hence the importance of ensuring a good supply of essential fats in the diet (see Essential building blocks, pages 16–19). As children of this age use up their food rapidly, it is necessary to make sure that they are eating every two to three hours to keep their blood-sugar levels constant – this applies to their mood as well as their physical energy. Children who tire easily may not be eating the correct balance of carbohydrates to protein, so take a look at The Food Pyramid (pages 20–23) to check the different categories of foods and the recommended balance at different ages.

Mental problems

As we have seen, the 'terrible twos' phase falls into this age bracket, although in truth many children do not experience this stage until their third or even fourth year – if at all. This phase usually refers to a tendency towards moodiness or tantrums, and mood swings may result from the frustrations experienced when the brain wants to do something that the body hasn't yet learned. Alternatively, boredom sets in easily at this age, and it is important to offer plenty of stimulation in different forms. Rather than expecting your child to sit quietly and paint or draw for long periods of time, try to set up different activities that will challenge her senses of sight, touch, smell, taste and hearing throughout the day, alternating between those activities that involve physical and mental skills.

Brain food is essential now, because literally thousands of new pieces of information are reaching the brain every day. Essential fats (found in nuts, seeds and their oils, and oily fish) are important mainstays in the diet and should be offered on a regular basis.

Problems	Solutions
Physical	
Aching bones	Increase the intake of essential fats (nuts, seeds and oily fish) and protein (chicken, meat, wholegrains and shellfish).
Sore muscles	Increase the intake of complex carbohydrates (such as wholegrain cereals, buckwheat pancakes and corn muffins) and offer plenty of vegetables.
Muscle cramps	Increase B vitamins and magnesium, found in wholegrain breads (rye and wheat), rice and green leafy vegetables; plus foods that are naturally salty, such as fish, ham and fermented soya products (vegetarian).
Twitching nerves	First, rule out any physical accidents; then ensure a good intake of essential fats, dairy produce and fish.
Bedwetting	Look at food sensitivities, or foods and drinks served in the evening or with the last meal of the day; reduce the sugar levels in drinks and foods, as this may be causing irritation to the bladder.
Mental	
Mood swings	Increase the regularity of meals, and include some protein with each meal to slow down the release of glucose and maintain good moods for a longer period. Avoid giving too many sweet treats.
Tantrums	Look at how much artificial sugar your child is eating, then reduce it, if necessary; explore the possibility of food sensitivities; keep a food diary to track food/mood patterns (see Allergies and intolerances, pages 64–9).
Excessive Sleepiness	Increase the regularity of meals; look at possible food sensitivities; ensure a minimum intake of simple carbohydrates, and eliminate all convenience foods, because additives may be causing the problem.

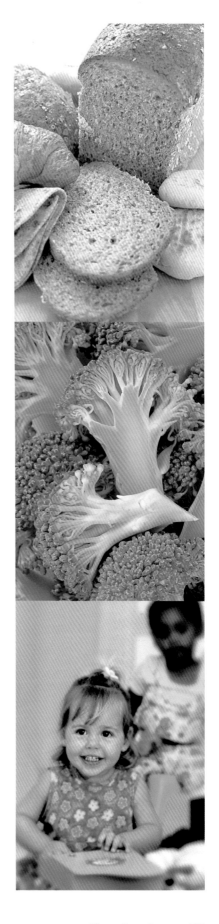

NOTE: Any problem not rectified *within a few days* of changing certain aspects of your child's diet indicates the possibility of another causal factor and you should seek medical advice.

Meal planners

By this age your child is eating full meals, including main courses and puddings, and will be having snacks in between. You can now use the whole of the recipe section, including the Essential main meals, choosing plenty of starch-based main courses, with proteins to balance. Good examples are Polenta Pizzas with a selection of toppings (see page 151), or pasta with meat or cheese sauces, such as Pasta Bows with Ham and Peas (see page 140) or Tuna Tagliatelle (see page 150).

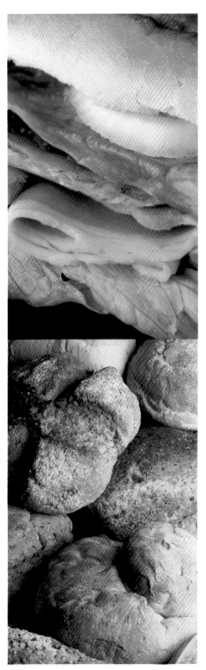

The inclusion of milk on a regular basis can be substituted by other forms of dairy produce (cheese, yoghurt or fromage frais), as your child eats more to obtain the required nutritional factors. If your child is dairy intolerant, or appears to shy away from such products, you can instead use rice milk, oat or soya milk, Yofu (soya yoghurt) and soya-based ice cream. For treats and puddings, it is perfectly possible to make ice cream at home (providing you have a proper ice cream maker, and follow the instructions carefully, storing the ice cream for no longer than five to six days as it will not have the preservatives that commercial ice-creams must carry). You can use oat or soya milk in place of cow's milk to make ice creams, and the advantage is that you can use fresh fruit purées to flavour the ice cream rather than highly sweetened artificial flavourings.

Yummy snacks and quick bites

For those families who are constantly on the move with older children being delivered and collected from school, remember that your younger child may not always be able to wait for the next meal that is being served to his siblings. Children of this age group need to eat every three hours, so ensure that you never leave home without a selection of quick bites and healthy foods, to avoid the temptation of buying salty or sweet ready-packed snacks.

I usually suggest to mothers that they treat their car as a second kitchen, always taking with them a couple of pieces of fruit, such as apples and bananas; some cheese bites or chunks cut from a larger piece of Cheddar or Edam; raw vegetable sticks; and flavoured rice cakes or oat cakes. These are all healthy between-meal snacks, depending on your child's preferences. Add to these a tub of hummus or avocado guacamole, either home-made or bought from the deli section of your supermarket, or a home-made 'whizzie' (see pages 148–9) and you have a well-balanced mini-meal.

One-week chart 18 months to 3 years

DAY 1

Breakfast	Brainy Seed Granola Cereal (see page 135). Glass of fruit juice, diluted 50 per cent with water
Mid-morning	Pear or plum
Lunch	Salmon fishcakes, carrots, peas and mashed or new potatoes. Fruit purée with fromage frais or soya yoghurt
Mid-afternoon	Oatcakes with nut butter or Marmite
Supper	Beany-Burgers (see page 138) with rice and mixed stir-fried vegetables. Ice cream. Glass of milk

DAY 2

Breakfast	Fluffy Scrambled Eggs (see page 136) with rye toast fingers. Apricot or nectarine. Glass of milk
Mid-morning	Yoghurt with honey and chopped fruit
Lunch	Chicken with Honeyed Vegetable Stir-Fry (see page 140). Glass of diluted juice
Mid-afternoon	Whizzie (see pages 148–9) with raw vegetable sticks or guacamole
Supper	Orzo with Creamy Mushroom Salsa (see page 150). Fruit. Glass of milk

DAY 3

Breakfast	Oaty Fruity Porridge (see page 134). Glass of milk
Mid-morning	Fromage frais with puréed fruit
Lunch	Tuna Tagliatelle (see page 150) with peas and baby sweetcorn. Glass of diluted fruit juice. Custardy Peaches and Bananas (see page 144)
Mid-afternoon	Carrot-Cake Muffin (see page 146). Glass of milk
Supper	Chicken with Rice (see page 142). Mixed Vegetable Mash (see page 139). Ice cream

DAY 4

Breakfast	Cornflakes with chopped banana and apple. Wholemeal toast with nut butter
Mid-morning	Date and Oat Flapjack (see page 145). Glass of milk
Lunch	Vegetable stir-fry with ham (or tofu). Apple Bomb (see page 145). Glass of diluted fruit juice. Piece of fruit
Mid-afternoon	Cup of popcorn (home-made!)
Supper	Beany Eggs on Rye (see page 151). Fruit Fool Flummery (see page 147)

DAY 5

Breakfast	Soaked Muesli with chopped mango or papaya. Glass of milk or small bio yoghurt with a little added honey
Mid-morning	Bunch of grapes and chunk of cheese
Lunch	Baked potato with grated cheese or salmon, mange tout and butternut squash (baked with potato). Home-made Ice-Lolly (see page 147). Glass of diluted fruit juice
Mid-afternoon	Date and Oat Flapjack (see page 145). Glass of milk
Supper	Polenta Pizza (see page 151) and mixed steamed vegetables with added butter

DAY 6

Breakfast	Poached eggs on wholemeal toast with slice of ham or mushrooms. Glass of diluted fruit juice. Piece of fruit
Mid-morning	Two rice cakes or Ryvita with Marmite or Vegemite. Glass of milk
Lunch	Baked beans with sausages (meat or vegetarian) with mashed potatoes and peas or French beans. Fruit Fool Flummery (see page 147). Glass of diluted fruit juice
Mid-afternoon	Chickpea and Green Pesto Whizzie (see page 149) with corn chips or carrot and celery sticks
Supper	Chicken stir-fry with mixed vegetables and rice. Fruity Rice Pudding (see page 146)

DAY 7

Breakfast	Buckwheat Pancakes (see page 136) with honey and sliced fresh fruit. Plain bio yoghurt. Glass of milk or diluted fruit juice
Mid-morning	Carrot-Cake Muffin (see page 146)
Lunch	Roast chicken with roasted parsnips and sweet potatoes, stir-fried mixed vegetables. Apple or rhubarb crumble with fromage frais. Glass of milk
Mid-afternoon	Piece of fruit or popcorn
Supper	Baked potato with grated cheese and tomato passata, or Chicken and Lentil Soup (see page 137) and wholemeal bread. Glass of diluted fruit juice. Small bunch of grapes

Nutrients for development

B-complex vitamins
Choline
Folic acid
Iron
Omega-3
Omega-6
Selenium
Vitamin A
Vitamin C
Vitamin E
Zinc

At this stage your child will be attending nursery or primary school on a regular basis, learning new social skills and acquiring a huge variety of new information. Foods to feed the brain are essential, but so too are those that help to boost the immune system, as your child will be faced with all manner of viruses and infections.

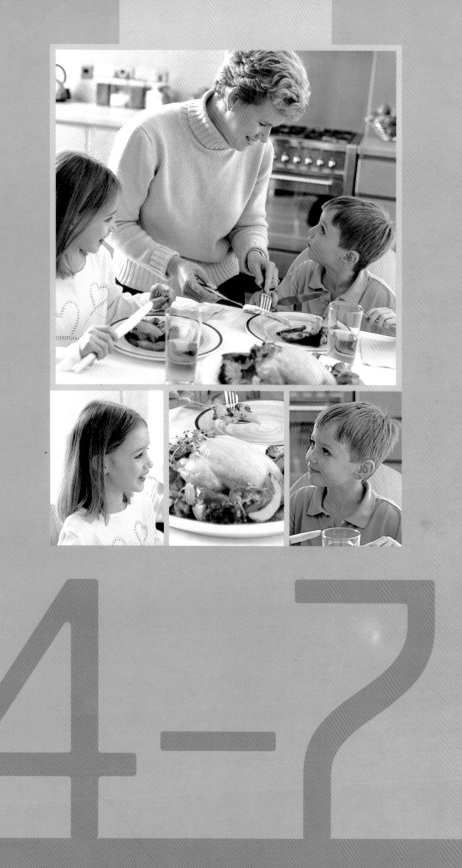

4-7

4 to 7 years

Stages of development

Your child's immune system is always important, and it is probably one of the most complex systems in the body, which works round the clock every day that we are alive. Approaching your child's immunity through his diet is the best place to start.

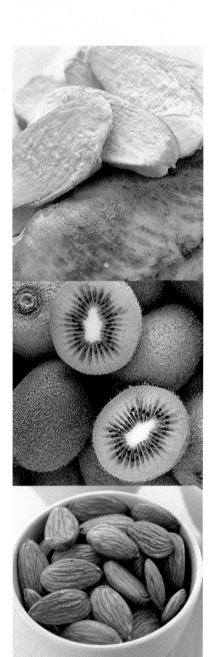

Bug-fighting and immunity

Congregating with other children in school on a daily basis presents one of the first major challenges to your child's immune system, as common bugs and bacterial infections run riot in school classrooms, dining halls and play areas. While all schools will encourage unwell children to be kept at home to avoid mass infection, some parents believe that their children are better off being exposed to colds and infections to increase their immunity.

Neither approach is necessarily incorrect, but some children are stronger than others, and there is no point in forcing your child to go to school if he has a temperature and is obviously unwell. Developing a sensitivity for when he is genuinely ill, as opposed to reluctant, is important.

The role of zinc and selenium

These two minerals are needed for the development of the immune system as a whole. From the moment a mother goes into labour, almost her entire zinc reserves are passed through the placenta to her unborn child to prepare him for the immune challenges that await from the moment he is born.

Children who suffer from regular colds, coughs and other infections, or those who do not heal quickly when cut or bruised, may be deficient in zinc, so ensure that adequate zinc-rich foods form a daily part of your child's diet. Zinc is found in all meats and poultry, egg yolks, sardines and tuna, oily fish and shellfish, oats, rye, buckwheat and brown rice, as well as walnuts, almonds and sunflower seeds.

Selenium is required in much smaller doses, but is no less important, as it works with vitamin E to protect against bacteria and viruses and to neutralize toxins in the body. One of the easiest ways of determining a potential selenium deficiency is by the frequency of colds, chest and other infections, as selenium is an important antioxidant required by the immune system. The richest sources of selenium are seafood and shellfish, sesame seeds, brazil nuts and wheatgerm.

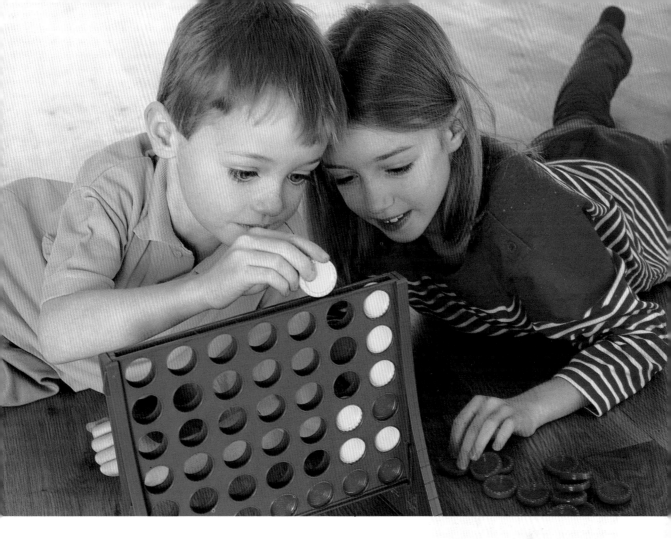

ACE vitamins: natural protectors

We all know that vitamin C is vital to the immune system, but so too are vitamins A and E. All work together in protecting the body from bacterial infections and viruses, and should be derived from foods eaten on a daily basis.

Humans cannot store vitamin C, so it is essential to eat foods such as citrus and kiwi fruits, red berries, green leafy vegetables, peppers, potatoes, sweet potatoes, broccoli and cabbage. Drinking large quantities of commercial citrus-based juices to obtain vitamin C is not ideal, as much of the vitamin C is lost from them, because they contain so much added sugar.

Vitamin A is found in two forms: animal (retinol) and vegetable (beta-carotene). Both are important to children, although they absorb it more easily in animal form, so vegetarian children need to eat plenty of beta-carotene, which is then converted into vitamin A. The best animal sources include liver, egg yolks, dairy produce and oily fish such as sardines and mackerel. Vegetable sources include leafy green vegetables, carrots (the beta-carotene gives them their bright orange colour), sweet potatoes, pumpkins and squashes, orange peppers, tomatoes, peaches, mangoes and papaya.

When all is not well

- Loss of appetite
- Quiet or subdued attitude
- Lack of concentration
- Apparent lethargy and an inability to 'get started'
- Crying for no apparent reason
- Temperature
- Dizziness, nausea or upset stomach
- Dry mouth and excessive thirst
- Pale, dry (or damp) skin

By the time your child is four years old, she will have developed the greatest part of her immune army (that part known as the IgG antibodies) to adult levels. From the age of about six months she will have started to develop her own antibodies (up until this point she relied on those passed on to her from her mother), and in the ensuing period the full quota has been developed. IgG antibodies make up almost 75 per cent of all antibodies found in the body and are vital for a strong immune system. They are responsible for protecting your child from viruses and bacteria, and for neutralizing toxins in the body.

Symptoms of anaemia

- Constant fatigue
- Physical weakness
- Pale skin (particularly on the face)
- Very pale inside lower eyelid
- Crying frequently
- Greater sensitivity to the cold
- Poor memory
- Frequent colds and infections

Vitamin E is found in the essential fatty acids in oily fish, and in nuts, seeds and their oils. Its main function is to protect all cells in the body from the damage of oxidation (like a cut apple turning brown when exposed to light and air), and to maintain soft, supple skin.

Iron-clad immunity

Iron is also vital for the immune system – it is required for the production of white blood cells in the immune army, and for creating the red blood cells that carry oxygen and nutrients in the bloodstream to every organ. If your child has a tendency to anaemia, it is important to know that there are three nutrients involved in this deficiency-related problem: iron, folic acid and vitamin B12.

Vegetarian (and vegan) children have a greater risk of becoming anaemic, because B12 is derived primarily from animal-based foods such as liver, beef and pork, fish and shellfish (and eggs, milk and cheese). Iron is also more available to children in animal form (such as liver, red meat and eggs), although it is found in many fruits and vegetables (including peaches, figs and apricots, cherries, bananas and avocados), as well as brown rice, potatoes and broccoli. Folic acid is most abundant in dark-green leafy vegetables, egg yolks, apricots, avocados, and wholewheat and rye grains. It is possible to give your child all three nutrients in a bountiful breakfast of muesli, fresh and dried fruits, and milk or yoghurt. Especially beneficial is giving your child green vegetables with fruit high in vitamin C, for example broccoli and orange juice, as this increases the bio-availability of iron.

Bigger brains – bigger appetite

At this age your child is starting to be challenged at an academic level, as well as physically in sport and games and in developing social skills. This introduces hundreds of new words, concepts and thoughts on a daily basis, and it is understandable that your child needs a wide range of foods to help with such rapid brain development.

The main nutrients required now are the essential fats found in oily fish, nuts, seeds and their oils, and the B-complex vitamins – especially choline, which is essential for the connection of thought processes. Choline can be found in most green leafy vegetables (as can other B vitamins), wheatgerm and egg yolks, as well as liver.

Teatime tiredness

If you have already become aware of your child's need for frequent meals, you will witness this even more dramatically when he comes home from school. It is usually at this time of day that blood-sugar levels are at their lowest, when your child is tired and may have eaten nothing since lunchtime. Giving him a high-protein snack on the way home, or as soon as he arrives, will prevent arguments over teatime food and menu choices.

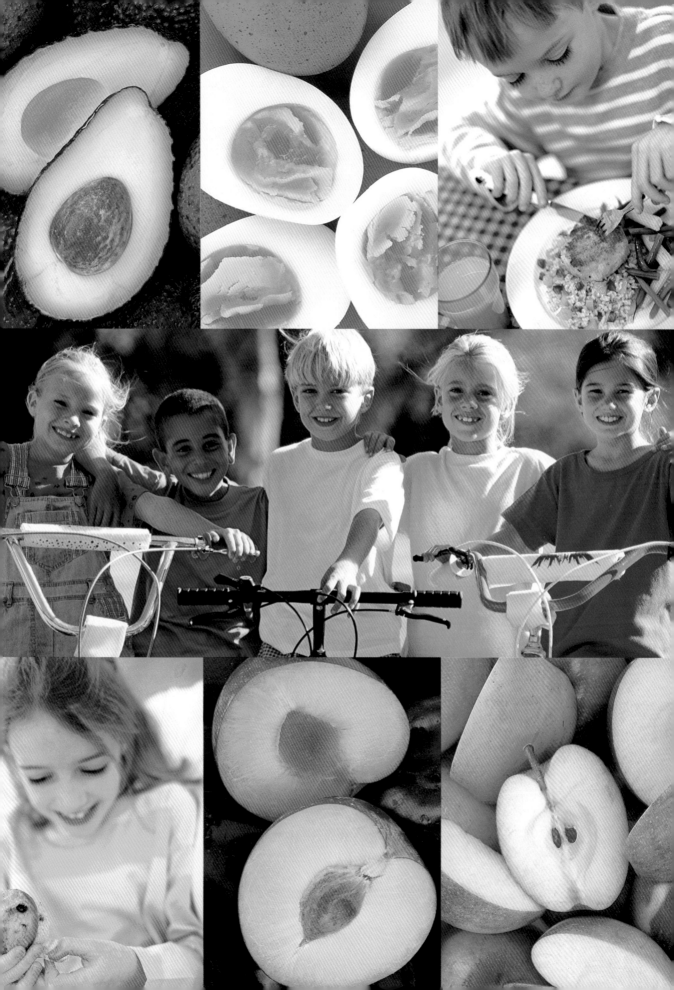

First school days

Big changes occur when your child first goes to kindergarten school, as a stricter regime has to be observed and the importance of breakfast becomes more apparent. Some children are not natural early risers, and the first school runs can present them with quite a challenge.

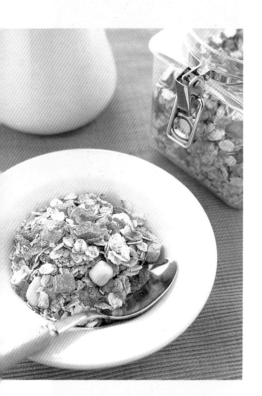

Meal planning

As most early activities revolve around group play and joint learning, rather than concentrating on the individual, the focus is on how well your child integrates with other children. However, as he progresses through this age group, his individual learning strengths or difficulties start to emerge and it is important to make sure that he is optimally fed at home, since he may not be getting all that he needs during school hours. Children with specific allergies and intolerances are sometimes better off taking their own foods to school to ensure a well-balanced eating regime. The Meal planners (pages 116–17) offer suggestions for healthy lunch boxes, as well as emphasizing meals at the beginning and end of the day, to create a better balance.

Peer pressure

It may seem unlikely that peer pressure will play a part in the eating choices of your child at this age, but the contrary is true. As your child makes friends and follows a specific group of children who appear to be like-minded in interests and upbringing, you may find that she starts coming home with out-of-the-ordinary questions about food and diet. It is best to be open and to keep your personal views to a minimum – it may be that your child has a good friend who is a vegetarian, and doesn't understand the reasons for such a choice. Exploring the subject with her is less likely to lead to fad-eating in the future than dismissing her questions as 'ridiculous'. This is an important area of your child's learning and social-skills development, particularly in multi-racial schools where many of the food choices relate to religion or social beliefs and restrictions.

Children often find school food unpalatable compared with home cooking, but the reality is that your child needs to eat during the day. Unless the school actively encourages parents to send lunch boxes and pre-packed foods, it is best to encourage him to eat some – if not all – of what is served at meal times. This can be a tricky stage, leading to restricted eating and the potential for food issues later on, so it is important to address problems as they arise and not to dismiss your child's concerns as 'inevitable'.

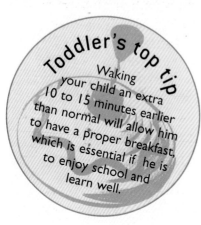

Toddler's top tip

Waking your child an extra 10 to 15 minutes earlier than normal will allow him to have a proper breakfast, which is essential if he is to enjoy school and learn well.

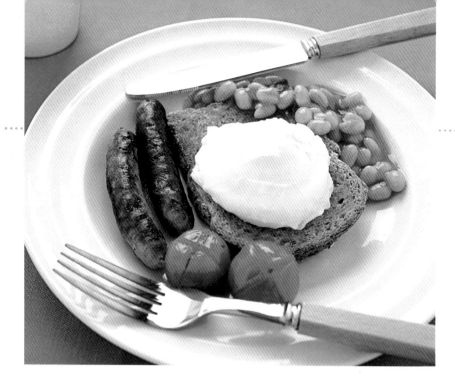

Fashionable diets are becoming more talked about at a younger age than ever before, because so much is now seen on television or discussed among parents. Take care not to impose your own dietary restrictions on your children at this young age, and take time to explain why another child's restrictions aren't necessarily suitable for them. It is common for children of this age to collectively cut out foods deemed 'too fatty' or 'disgusting', as they feel stronger in a herd than complaining individually. Make sure your child hasn't decided that he suddenly dislikes a food just because his best friend has, especially if you have always eaten it at home and it's healthy.

Big breakfasts and high teas

The start of the day and returning from school are the times when you are best able to ensure that your child is well nourished. As the morning is often a rush and there is the whole family to take care of, the best breakfasts are often prepared the previous night. Children should not feel rushed into eating the first meal of the day – if necessary, wake them 15–30 minutes earlier to ensure they have adequate time to eat a decent breakfast. A piece of toast and marmalade is not sufficient for children of this age – they will digest and use up the nutrients almost before they reach school.

Having choices available is also important: fruit salad, muesli or porridge, and a piece of toast with

Marmite or cream cheese, or yoghurt with honey, fruit and nuts make ideal uncooked options. Save eggs for the weekend if time really does not permit, but for those children who need a greater level of protein (such as those engaged in regular active sport), or prior to tests or recitals, it only takes a few minutes to whisk up scrambled eggs on wholewheat toast, and your child will be well set up for the day ahead.

If the journey to school lasts more than a few minutes, take a couple of pieces of fruit along that are safe to eat in the car, such as bananas or apples, particularly if your child has not eaten much breakfast.

Teatime should be organized so that your child can have her main meal of the day at this point. This may require some organization, especially if you are working. Using a slow-cooker or steamer allows foods to be cooked at a low temperature over the course of the whole day without damaging their nutritional content, and requires only the addition of rice or potatoes and fresh vegetables when you get home. All types of foods can be prepared in this way, from soups to casseroles containing meat or vegetarian alternatives.

Whilst pasta is quick and easy, it provides only a limited source of nutrients, and care should be taken to add a complex sauce to make up the largest part of the nutritional content. Rather than a simple tomato sauce, add chicken, ham, meat or beans and other pulses to a basic passata (strained tomato sauce) to provide a 'whole' meal. Alternatively, use a cheese-based sauce to which you add ham, mushrooms or beans to create a well-rounded dish. Serve it with vegetables, as this is the only meal when your child is likely to benefit from fresh vegetables.

Problems and solutions

Unfortunately, despite rigorous kitchen hygiene rules, food poisoning can occur at school and knowing how to recognize the signs is vital.

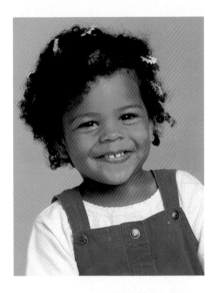

Food bugs and poisons

Food poisoning in young children can be serious, because vomiting and diarrhoea can dehydrate the body very rapidly, upsetting the delicate balance of minerals that regulate the body's functions (see Allergies and intolerances, pages 64–7). Food poisoning is not related to allergenic foods – it may be a result of food that is not fresh, or food that has been defrosted and insufficiently heated to kill off potential pathogens.

Taking packed lunches to school presents its own set of problems, as your child is unlikely to eat the contents within three or four hours of you packing the foods up. Ensure that all necessary foods are refrigerated until the last minute at home, and that lunch boxes are left in a relatively cool place at school (usually in an unheated corridor).

Common food bugs

- Campylobacter: now the most common of all food bacteria causing poisoning; most commonly found in chicken, meat and shellfish; can cause severe stomach cramps and nausea.
- Salmonella: considered to be the most virulent bug, although thankfully not the most common; causes severe diarrhoea, dramatic loss of fluid and possibly a raised temperature, sweating and dizziness; may be caught from under-cooked chicken or eggs, or salads and cooked foods left unrefrigerated for several hours; medical help should be sought immediately if salmonella is suspected.
- Bacillus cereus: typically found in cooked rice that has been kept warm or improperly reheated; it is important to eat rice as soon as it is cooked, or to refrigerate it as soon as it

has cooled down; this bacteria causes severe vomiting and/or diarrhoea, but is fortunately not long-lasting.
- Staphylococcus aureus: most frequently found in cream- and custard-filled pastries and cakes, or in ham and chicken; does not usually cause severe symptoms, although diarrhoea is the most prevalent one.
- Listeria: usually found in soft cheeses, ice cream and pre-packed ready-cooked meals; causes diarrhoea, vomiting and sweating.
- Escherichia coli (E. coli): most commonly found in hamburgers and other beef products that have been insufficiently cooked; can cause severe diarrhoea and spread undetected in schools and restaurants that do not observe the strictest hygiene codes.

Suggested remedies

Problems	Solutions
Frequent colds and infections	Identify the specific causes of a lowered immune system – increase fresh fruit and vegetables in the diet, and reduce the sugars from cola drinks and other fast foods that may be interfering with the absorption of nutrients; look at possible food intolerances that may be causing runny noses and blocked ears, such as dairy products, excess wheat-based foods or eggs.
Food poisoning/ diarrhoea	Give water only, restrict all food intake other than dry toast or rice crackers, and seek medical attention immediately; symptoms should not be allowed to continue for longer than 3–4 hours unattended.
Listlessness, fatigue, excessive sleeping	Check for anaemia (pale skin and other symptoms, see page 110); increase the intake of foods rich in iron, folic acid and B12, for maximum improvement: green leafy and orange vegetables, dried fruits, fish, shellfish, liver and eggs.
Poor concentration	Look at possible food sensitivities that may be upsetting blood-sugar levels. Ensure sufficient essential fats in the diet, for optimum cognitive function: increase the intake of oily fish, sunflower and pumpkin seeds (these may be ground and added to porridge). Increase the variety of wholegrains to provide the wide range of B-complex vitamins required for the brain and nervous system; also protein from animal or vegetable sources, to stimulate the transmission of information.
Physical weakness, loss of stamina	Check eating habits to ensure the regular consumption of meals. Increase complex carbohydrate intake for several days until energy has returned to normal levels. Check bowel habits to ensure that food is being properly digested and absorbed. Increase the intake of B-complex vitamins to provide the nutrients for energy production: porridge oats, muesli mixes, rye crackers, brown rice, green leafy vegetables, fish, chicken and eggs.

The not-eating syndrome

Observing how your child is performing at school, and how tired he is when he comes home, will give you a fairly accurate measure of how much he is, or is not, eating. Whether refusing to eat is due to insufficient choice or quality at school, or to the habits of friends and classmates, is irrelevant – your child will not be able to sustain his concentration, focus and memory if he is not eating during the day. Understanding the reasons is essential, but a solution needs to be arrived at through discussions with your child and/or the school.

Try to determine if a not-eating phase is due to something else that is happening at school: if your child is being bullied or left out of the mainstream, this will affect her appetite. So too will teasing (if, say, she is heavier than most of the others), and this will be the fastest way towards an altered attitude to food.

Can't concentrate/fidgeting

It is at this age that the first signs of possible hyperactivity may become apparent. If your child has always been very active and even a little disruptive at home, this will be highlighted in a school environment, where the discipline of sitting still in a classroom may become impossible, and you should seek the help of a doctor or other specialist. Look at Recognizing hyperactivity (pages 70–71) to see if the symptoms seem familiar – your child may have an acute sensitivity to foods or additives and chemicals that he is consuming regularly, and this needs to be identified before his behaviour is likely to change.

Meal planners

By this age your child is eating regular, full meals, and probably requires four per day, rather than three. I suggest that children in school should have a light tea when they come home, and supper, but where this isn't practical ensure that you take some pieces of fruit, mixed nuts or seed and oat bars to greet them with. Children at this age are often exhausted by the end of their school day, and usually ravenously hungry. It is little wonder that so many tetchy words are exchanged in car rides on the way home!

Sandwich fillings:

Wholegrain pitta pockets offer a much healthier option than the standard white sandwich loaf.

- Ham with lettuce, cucumber, (optional alfalfa sprouts on top) and mayonnaise
- Chicken slices with sundried tomato pesto
- Cream cheese with watercress or baby spinach leaves, and sliced tomatoes
- Humus with mixed sprouted seeds (vegetarian option)
- Tuna mixed with a little crème fraiche, chopped cucumber or shredded lettuce
- Thinly sliced turkey with cranberry sauce and chopped red pepper.
- Sliced cheddar or edam/emmenthal cheese with rocket, watercress or lettuce.

Experiment with what you have available in the fridge and invite your child to make up some of his own combinations.

Handing your child sweets or a chocolate bar when he finishes school may elevate his spirits momentarily, but you will find it much more difficult to get him to sit down and concentrate on any homework projects as his blood sugar levels will drop 20 to 30 minutes later.

Fresh fruits and raw vegetable sticks are ideal for the car, together with some fromage frais or a whizzie (see pages 148–9). Make sure your child eats it while the car is stationary to avoid the risk of choking.

Lively lunch box combos

Many schools require lunches to be supplied by the parents. There is now a huge selection of brightly-coloured, attractive, ready-prepared lunch boxes which are all, sadly, full of highly salted and/or sugary snack foods, which only contribute to an increase in hyperactive types of behaviour. What your child needs is a fully nutritious meal in the middle of the day to keep him going throughout the afternoon.

The key to a successful lunch box is to have a selection of three or four different items, to tease the eyes and tastebuds, as well as providing a full range of nutrients. You may wish to pre-pack most of the ingredients in the box the night before and keep it fresh in the fridge.

Key ingredients:

Piece of fruit: apples, bananas, pears, firm peaches or nectarines, apricots, oranges or satsumas are all suitable fruits that won't get damaged or squashed in a lunch box.

Raw vegetable sticks: carrots, celery, red and green bell peppers, small cucumbers, baby tomatoes, baby sweetcorn, small asparagus spears, french beans with dips and whizzies (see pages 148–9).

Sandwich: Children love the appearance of a halved pitta stuffed with goodies of their own choosing (see left).

For a change: Soups (e.g. chicken noodle or Tuscan bean), bio yoghurts with a dash of honey, creme caramel or rice pudding.

One-week chart 4 to 7 years

DAY 1

Breakfast Muesli with natural yoghurt or Rice Dream rice milk (soak overnight in 50 per cent apple juice and 50 per cent water to enhance natural sweetness), and add yoghurt or dairy alternative, and fresh fruits of choice. Glass of fresh fruit juice diluted 50 per cent with water

Lunch Shepherd's pie with peas and broccoli or Bean Pot with wholegrain bread (see page 138). Piece of fruit, or natural yoghurt with fruit purée.

Mid afternoon Cottage or cream cheese on slice of rye bread with small bunch of grapes

Supper Tuna Tagliatelle (see page 150) or pasta with lentil and tomato sauce for vegetarians. Custardy Peaches and Bananas (see page 144)

DAY 2

Breakfast Fluffy Scrambled Eggs (see page 136) or boiled eggs with wholemeal toast (cut into fingers for the younger child). Extra toast with Marmite or Vegemite, or low-sugar marmalade (e.g. St. Dalfour). Glass of milk or diluted fruit juice

Lunch Baked potato and tuna (may be tinned) with carrots and courgettes. Pear with vanilla ice cream

Mid-afternoon 1 cup popcorn (home-made preferably with no added sugar.

Supper Orzo with Creamy Mushroom Salsa (see page 150)

DAY 3

Breakfast Oaty Fruity Porridge (see page 134) with chopped fresh fruit and blanched almonds (soak porridge overnight in milk or water to reduce cooking time). Glass of diluted fruit juice

Lunch Macaroni cheese (wholewheat pasta) or Chicken and Lentil Soup (see page 137) with wholemeal bread. Piece of fruit

Mid afternoon Nut butter (almond or cashew) on rice crackers or toast

Supper Beany-Burgers (see page 138) with sweetcorn and rice. Apple bombs (see page 145)

DAY 4

Breakfast Baked beans (low-sugar variety) on wholemeal toast. Glass of milk

Lunch Chicken (or tofu) with Rice (see page 142). Bio yoghurt with fresh fruit and honey

Mid afternoon Carrot-Cake Muffin (see page 146)

Supper Fisherman's Pasta Bake (see page 141). Fruit

DAY 5

Breakfast Cornflakes with chopped banana and raisins. Wholemeal toast and Marmite or Vegemite. Glass of diluted fruit juice

Lunch Polenta Pizza with toppings of choice (see page 151). Fruity Rice Pudding (see page 146)

Tea Yoghurt with fruit or Brainy Seed Granola Bar (see page 135)

Supper Sticky Lamb Cutlets (see page 142), or marinated tempeh for vegetarians, with butternut squash purée and French fries.

DAY 6

Breakfast Rice and Fruit Compote (see page 135). Glass of diluted fruit juice, piece of wholemeal toast and marmalade

Lunch Pasta Bows with Ham and Peas (see page 140), Home-made Ice-Lolly (see page 147)

Mid afternoon Kidney Bean, Tomato and Mustard Whizzie (see page 149) and fresh vegetable sticks

Supper Beany Eggs on Rye (see page 151). Ice cream or soya ice cream

DAY 7

Breakfast Carrot-Cake Muffin (see page 146). Fromage frais. Glass of diluted fruit juice

Lunch Almost-Adult Beef Curry (see page 143). Fruit Fool Flummery (see page 147)

Mid-afternoon Piece of fresh fruit and Date and Oat Flapjacks (see page 145)

Supper Pitta pocket sandwich (see opposite). Milkshake (use fresh fruit in blender)

Nutrients for development

Biotin
Boron
Calcium
Essential fats
Magnesium
Manganese
Selenium
Vitamin E
Zinc

This exciting stage transforms your child into a young adult, with rapid changes in the sexual hormonal systems, as well as huge demands on their brain development, social skills and physical activity. Eating like an adult allows your child the full range of foods and nutrients that he or she needs to adapt in all these areas of development.

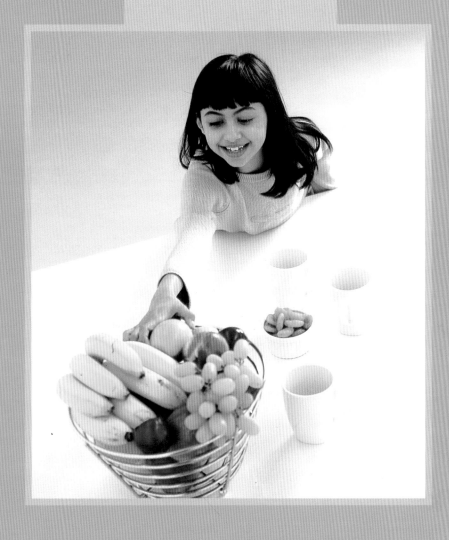

8→

8 years to puberty

Stages of development

The transition from young child to young adult appears to happen overnight. How many times have you heard a parent exclaim, 'It must have happened in his sleep'. Most growth and repair does indeed take place when we are asleep (one of the reasons why adequate sleep is so important), but the transformation from child to adult does happen rapidly.

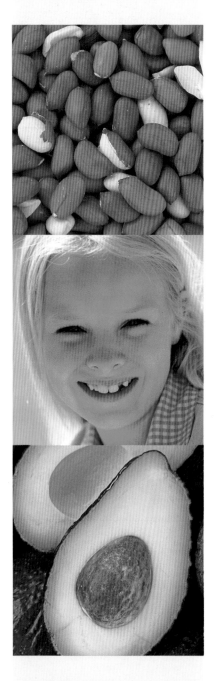

From little to large

Perhaps the most obvious change is in shape or height. Growth occurs in spurts, but these do not happen at set times – to the frustration of siblings who are close in age, with the younger sometimes being taller than the elder. Late physical developers are not necessarily immature in mind and intellect – it is their hormones that determine when they change from child to young adult.

A youngster of eight years is still very much a child, but that same child may develop primary and secondary sexual organs within two years, with some girls experiencing their first menstruation at nine or 10. While this is still rare, it seems that the age of sexual maturity is occurring at a younger age than it did, say, 50 years ago, although the reason is not clearly understood.

Hormone mayhem

The development of the sex organs can occur very rapidly, and many children will start covering up their bodies as breasts start to emerge and male genitalia become more obvious.

In a young man, the first sign of sexual development is usually the appearance of sporadic facial, pubic and body hair. It is important not to draw too much attention to this, to avoid causing excessive self-consciousness in your child – remember that he is probably trying to come to terms with these changes. In addition, his voice may start to break, a transition that rarely occurs smoothly, causing embarrassment to the child and fond amusement to the all-knowing parents.

In young girls, changes in body shape – including greater roundness to the hip area and enlargement of the breasts – occur, with pubic and underarm hair appearing around the same time. In girls who start menstruation early, changes in body shape and size tend to happen quickly, whereas those who start their periods later often remain more immature in shape well into their teenage years. In a small number of girls, the onset of menstruation is unusually painful, especially in those whose mothers have experienced hormone-related problems, such as fibroids, endometriosis or polycystic ovarian syndrome (PCOS). Seek medical help if you are concerned that your child is experiencing particularly severe symptoms for one so young. Remember that heavy menstruation may lead to temporary iron deficiency.

Emotional roller-coasters

As fast as the physical changes are taking place, so is the emotional roller-coaster ride. This is the first of several major transitions in an adult's life, and isn't always easy. If your child suddenly becomes stubborn, argumentative, uncompromising or downright difficult, you may want to question whether this is due to sexual development, rather than simply standing up for himself. Explaining what is happening to him from your own perspective may help to keep the communication channels open.

Food for thought

Such major upsets to the body's equilibrium inevitably cause dietary changes. You may find that your child starts to favour different foods – often choices that are not particularly healthy – and want to encourage better eating patterns, especially if a maturing child is putting on excessive weight or becoming uncomfortable about her size and shape. It may be easier to take her to see a nutritionist or other health-care practitioner, who can best explain the reasons for specific dietary choices in a more scientific way than a concerned parent.

Skin scourge

The faster the hormonal changes occur, the more likely your child is to have troubled skin, and this will be exacerbated by poor eating habits and excessive sugars in the diet. A minimal amount of skin eruptions and oiliness is normal; full-blown acne is not, and can cause enormous psychological problems. Rather than trying a myriad of commercially advertised remedies, look at the causes of such a scourge.

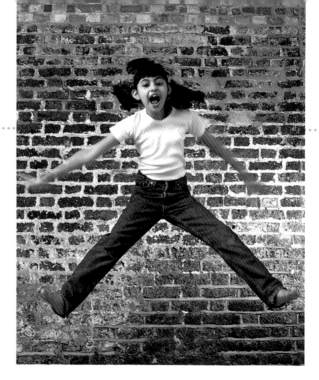

Diet can play a large part in improving even the worst skin problems, particularly if there are foods to which your child may have an intolerance. Culprits include dairy products, citrus fruits and eggs, aside from all the obvious sugared foods and those with additives and colourings. If your child was sensitive to foods at a young age, experiencing eczema or other skin problems, then food is likely to be one of the main causes, although not necessarily the only one. Evaluation of such foods can offer an immediate improvement and prevent years of self-consciousness. Another major consideration is zinc deficiency (see Grown-up food, pages 122–3).

Bones and structure

As your child goes through major changes in shape and size, so does the structure of her bones. At this stage, bones are reaching maturity, and the inclusion of plenty of bone-building nutrients is vital.

Children often complain of what parents call 'growing pains', but which are more specifically the building of bone density. It is important for your child to be physically active, and research shows that a high percentage of children get less than one hour of exercise per day. Strong bones are built on weight-bearing exercise, and sitting in front of a computer or television is not going to help, so encourage your child to engage in a variety of games that allow him to use his growing body constructively.

Grown-up food

By this stage, meals served to your children need be no different than those you prepare for yourself, and family meals should have become commonplace whenever possible. Your child's appetite may well exceed your own, particularly during a growth spurt, and large, healthy appetites should be encouraged to support this period of rapid development at several levels.

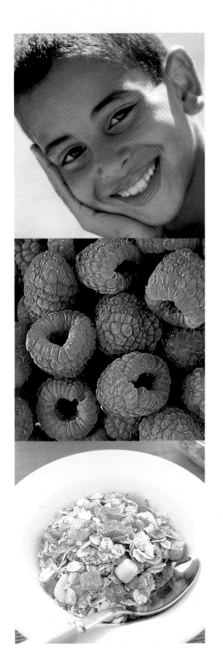

The importance of fats in the diet

Essential fats are vital for the development of the sexual organs and for hormone production, as well as for ensuring soft and supple skin. Children on very low-fat diets may have their development delayed or complicated without the parent being aware of the effects of this kind of restriction. The saturated fats found in packet crisps, bacon bits and other such snacks interfere with the utilization of beneficial fats, and children will often crave these fats at this time, without realizing that their body is actually yearning for the healthier alternative.

Fish in any form is also crucial at this point, and if your child has not favoured fish up to now, he may benefit from the same type of essential fats from nuts, seeds and their oils. Including a variety of nuts and seeds in breakfast cereals, or mixed in with yoghurt and fruit compotes, is an excellent way of ensuring that some of these essential fats are eaten. Many young girls tend to avoid nuts, fearing that they are excessively high in fat, without understanding their benefits. Both groups of foods are also rich sources of vitamin E, which is essential for good skin.

No to low-fat diets

Another important consideration is that of weight gain at this age. If your child was prone to puppy fat at a younger age, she may expect to lose it now, only to find that her weight has increased with the onset of hormonal changes. Cutting fat completely from the diet in the hope of losing weight will only prove to be detrimental, as the essential fats are vital to ensure the removal of fat that is stored in the adipose tissues (areas of concentrated fat cells).

The zinc connection

Zinc is one of the most important minerals required by the body, and is used for more than 200 different enzyme functions. It is especially important for growth, for the development of the sexual organs and

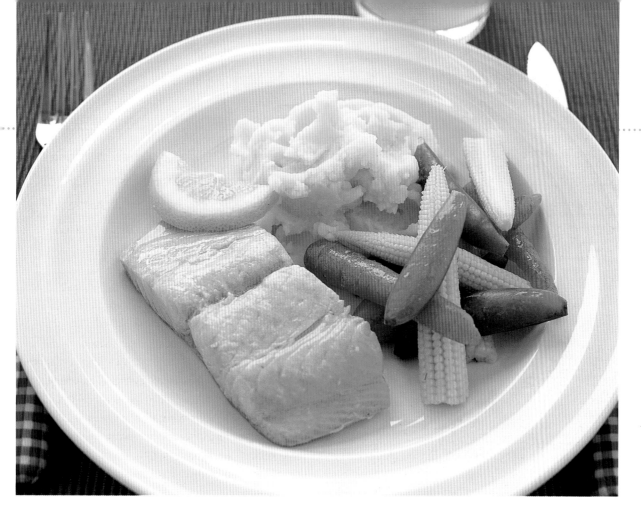

the production of sex hormones. Zinc deficiency is common in young adolescents, as their bodies use more than they are likely to consume on a regular daily basis. One telltale sign of zinc deficiency is white flecks in the fingernails, and with the onset of sperm production and male maturity, this is not uncommon, as sperm require zinc for their formation. Include plenty of red meat, chicken, fish and shellfish, which are all rich sources of zinc, or wholegrains, pulses, nuts and seeds in those who prefer a vegetarian diet.

As zinc is also vital for the repair and healing of all tissues in the body, skin health is dependent on good sources of this mineral. Skin that heals slowly or poorly will benefit from additional supplementation, as well as from daily sources of zinc-rich foods.

Vitamin C works in conjunction with zinc, so ensure that plenty of vitamin C-rich foods are included, such as red berry fruits, potatoes, broccoli and cabbage. Avoid citrus-fruit drinks if there is a skin problem, as citrus fruit tends to be one of the food groups that irritate and worsen the condition.

Perfect proteins

At this age many children, especially boys, desire a much higher proportion of red meat and other primary proteins. As proteins form the building blocks of all organs and tissues in the body, it is easy to understand why. However, encouraging the consumption of lean protein is preferable to offering meat that is high in fat content or quantities of fried foods, which may be satisfying to the palate, but are not as nutritious as their leaner, cleaner alternatives.

Since most proteins also contain abundant quantities of calcium (found in dairy foods, nuts, red meat, egg yolks and poultry), good supplies of these foods should be included in your meal plans to ensure the key nutrients for bone-mineral density. Magnesium, which is needed to absorb calcium into bone, is found primarily in wholegrains, pulses and green leafy vegetables. Children approaching adolescence often lack sufficient fresh vegetables in their diet, so including them in soups and sandwiches, or spreads and dips, is a good way of making sure that they are getting a daily supply.

Problems and solutions

The problems that occur during this age group relate mainly to growth and maturity, which may be either too fast or too slow, with the child finding himself set apart, or different, from his peers.

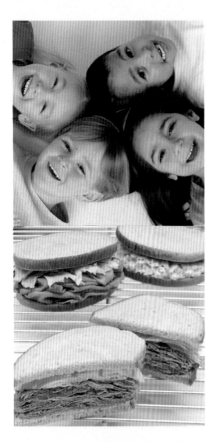

Limited diets

It seems ironic that, with all the choices available to us of foods from around the world, many people still have very limited diets. The advent of ready-prepared foods has changed our attitude towards cooking meals from scratch, and many children now have two parents who work full-time. Children are no longer taught domestic science at school, so they don't have an example of the taste and benefits of preparing fresh food. It is often cheaper to buy pre-packed dishes than all the component ingredients. And, with the growing popularity of online shopping, the temptation to see foods in the flesh is bypassed at the click of a button. All these factors contribute towards an attitude of eating as a means of survival, rather than for pleasure and family nourishment.

Good food, good mood

As your child approaches puberty, she will go through a myriad of emotional surges and dips. For those children on a highly refined diet of fast foods, this problem is likely to be exacerbated, causing irritability and aggression (see Sugar and spice, pages 38–41). A diet that is high in cola drinks, highly sugared cereals, cakes and snacks is also likely to have a detrimental effect on your child's concentration and school work. Sugars, as well as many artificial colourings, sweeteners and additives, can cross the blood-brain barrier, affecting the way your child perceives herself and others.

All hormones produced in the body work in tandem with others and so, if blood-sugar levels are repeatedly high, this has a knock-on effect, interfering with the delicate balance of the metabolism, sexual-organ development and stress management.

Good mood food requires that fresh foods should make up the greatest part of the diet, with at least one serving daily of essential fats from fish, nuts, seeds or their oils; nut butters deliver these in a practical, tasty way to children. A balance of proteins and complex carbohydrates at every meal and snack will ensure even blood-sugar levels, reducing the likelihood of sulking, irritability and off-handedness, which are often associated with the onset of adolescence.

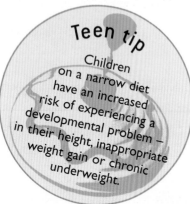

Teen tip

Children on a narrow diet have an increased risk of experiencing a developmental problem – in their height, inappropriate weight gain or chronic underweight.

Suggested remedies

Problems	Solutions
Mood swings, lack of concentration	Balance blood-sugar levels by increasing complex carbohydrates, fibre and protein, and reducing fast foods and sugars/sweets.
Excessive weight gain	Look at reasons for this: physical/hormonal and emotional. Regulate the diet by eliminating many of the processed or highly sugared foods, replacing them with the proteins found in chicken, fish, lean meat, eggs and moderate amounts of nuts and seeds. Consider hormonal influence on metabolic rate, and increase the amount of exercise your child is taking.
Underweight	Explore the possibility of dietary restrictions or not eating at school. Add more complex carbohydrates, to provide energy and muscle-building material; and some fats. Ensure she is eating regularly, even when away from home.
Shortness in height	Look at the amount of protein: increase dairy produce, eggs, poultry, meat, pulses, nuts and seeds. Add zinc and calcium/magnesium supplements on the advice of a nutritionist.
Rapid development of sexual organs	Ensure plenty of zinc-rich foods (see page 155); these are found in chicken, eggs, fish and shellfish, wholegrains, nuts and seeds, all of which also supply essential fats to help balance the hormones and maintain good skin.
Painful early periods	Magnesium relaxes the muscle cramps that cause painful periods; it is found in all green leafy vegetables, almonds, figs, tomatoes, garlic, onions and chicken, plus high cocoa-content chocolate (in moderation).
Spotty skin/acne	Zinc is vital for healing the skin and tissue below the surface, as well as reducing the acne caused by hormonal changes. Cleanse the diet of all salty, high-sugar snacks and fast foods; look at dairy food, tomatoes and citrus fruits as possible food intolerances (high acidity); increase the water intake to 1.5 litres (2½ pt) per day and avoid concentrated fruit juices.
Excessive body hair in girls	Have hormone levels tested by a doctor – this is usually an indication of an imbalance, which may need to be addressed with medication.
Unexplained fatigue	Check for sufficient variety in the diet and provide B vitamins for energy, from wholegrain cereals and rice, green leafy vegetables, fish, yoghurt, cheese, lean meat, chicken and eggs.

Skin deep

As hormone changes are likely to bring about spots and even acne at this time, it is worth drawing attention to skin care and maintenance at an early stage. No amount of creams, lotions and potions is going to have the same curative effect as consuming plenty of fresh vegetables, some fruits and lots of water, while discouraging an excessive intake of chocolate, cola drinks and other sweet treats.

Antibiotics are often prescribed for more severe cases of acne, but this simply masks the problem and is upsetting to the digestive tract, as antibiotics kill off all bacteria in the intestines: good as well as bad. Looking into the possibility of food intolerances, or an imbalance of acid/alkaline, is a more appropriate first step and should reduce the severity of the problem to an acceptable level, without having to take medication.

Meal planners

Children are now growing up much faster than the last generation did, with many of them becoming more aware of the development of their own bodies at a far younger age. Young girls are setting aside their dolls by the time they are six or seven, and turning to the games and communication possibilities that are so readily available by mobile phones or personal computers. Television too allows them to watch people that are many years older than themselves, and they may start to emulate their behaviour.

Fridge Feasts

- Ham
- Chicken
- Lean sliced beef or cooked lamb
- Cheeses such as cheddar, edam, emmenthal, gouda and parmesan
- Cooked tuna or salmon fillets
- Shellfish – cooked shell-on prawns
- Smoked meats (to satisfy salt cravings)
- Yoghurt (plain bio)
- Fromage frais
- Nut butters
- Cooked lentil dishes (such as Indian dalh)

Cola drinks are out! They contain absolutely no goodness whatsoever. Instead why not combine some fresh apple, pear, cranberry, peach or mango juice with sparkling water.

Clean foods

In order to handle the secondary developmental problems of hormonal changes you need to ensure that your child does not start developing a craving for packet crisps and snacks, cola drinks and other popular fast food choices, as these are the culprits of spotty skin, weight gain and dramatic mood swings.

The rapid changes of hormones often lead to cravings for highly salted foods and quick-release energy foods. This is indicative of your child's needs for added zinc, as male and female hormonal development is particularly dependent on this mineral, found in protein foods such as shellfish, chicken and red meat and wholegrains. This is therefore a time for an increase in protein foods in the diet, rather than carbohydrates, as the body's physical and emotional changes are more noticeable now.

Soups

Not all children like soup but, if yours do, it is worth investing in a one-person size thermos to ensure that they have a hot part to their winter meal. Tomato is often a favourite, but is not enough on its own for a lunchtime meal. Try adding some kidney beans or chick peas and blend until smooth to add protein and bulk to this and other vegetable soups. Alternatively, chicken noodle soup, ham and pea, or Tuscan bean style soups offer a good balance of nutrients in one cup. Many of the freshly prepared soups in the supermarkets today are excellent, and are additive and preservative free.

Puddings

It is not necessary to provide a pudding every day. Encouraging your child to eat a piece of fruit as an alternative is a far better practice, but simple puddings may be included from time to time as a treat, rather than the norm. Blending plain bio yoghurt with some good quality honey and fresh fruit is easy to put together in the morning, and can be kept safely in the lunch box until lunch time in cool conditions.

DAY 1

Breakfast Fluffy Scrambled Eggs (see page 136) with wholemeal toast. Glass of diluted apple juice

Lunch Fisherman's Pasta Bake (see page 141) with green leaf salad. Poached or fresh peaches

Mid-afternoon Crackers with nut butter

Supper Beany-Burgers (see page 138), with Honeyed Vegetable Stir-Fry (see page 140)

Snack Avocado dip with raw vegetables

DAY 2

Breakfast Brainy Seed Granola Cereal (see page 135). Glass of diluted fruit juice

Lunch Lean slices of ham with tomato, avocado and watercress salad or pea and ham soup with wholemeal bread

Mid-afternoon Cottage cheese on rice crackers or raw apple slices

Supper Pasta Bows with Ham and Peas (see page 140), baby spinach or french beans. Fresh fruit salad

Snack Red Pepper and Butterbean Whizzie (see page 149) with raw vegetable sticks

DAY 3

Breakfast Smoothie with banana, mango or peach, almonds or walnuts, pumpkin and sunflower seeds, with milk and bio yoghurt (blended until smooth). Buckwheat Pancakes (see page 136)

Lunch Bean Pot (see page 138) with brown rice. Apple Bomb with fromage frais (see page 145)

Mid-afternoon Mixed dried fruit and nuts. Glass of diluted fruit juice

Supper Sticky Lamb Cutlets (see page 142) or tempeh/soya burgers, with Mixed Vegetable Mash (see page 139). Fruity Rice Pudding (see page 146)

Snack Fresh fruit

DAY 4

Breakfast Oaty Fruity Porridge (see page 134) with added nuts and seeds. Glass of juice

Lunch Beany Eggs on Rye (see page 151) with added slice of ham. Fruit Fool Flummery (see page 147)

Mid-afternoon Carrot-Cake Muffin (see page 146). Glass of milk

Supper Almost-Adult Beef Curry (see page 143) with rice and fresh vegetables. Piece of fruit

Snacks Crackers with nut butter

DAY 5

Breakfast Cornflakes or rice puffs with raisins, fromage frais and chopped apple. Wholemeal toast with low-sugar marmalade. Glass of diluted fruit juice

Lunch Orzo with Creamy Mushroom Salsa (see page 150), green salad and olive oil dressing

Mid-afternoon Date and Oat Flapjack (see page 145) and bunch of grapes

Supper Chicken tikka with rice and dalh, or vegetarian curry with rice, poppadoms. Fresh mango chutney

Snack Chickpea and Green Pesto Whizzie (see page 149) with raw vegetable sticks

DAY 6

Breakfast Two poached eggs on wholemeal toast with slice of ham or bacon, grilled tomatoes. Glass of milk or diluted fruit juice

Lunch Tuna Tagliatelle (see page 150). Home-made Ice-Lolly (see page 147)

Mid-afternoon Piece of fruit and handful of nuts

Supper Chicken and mixed vegetable casserole with mashed sweet potatoes and mangetout

Snack Date and Oat Flapjack (see page 145)

DAY 7

Breakfast Rice and Fruit Compote (see page 135). Glass of milk or milkshake with fresh fruit

Lunch Grilled prawns or grilled fillet of fish with mixed roasted root vegetables and rice

Mid-afternoon Carrot--Cake Muffin (see page 146)

Dinner Polenta Pizza (see page 151) with mixed salad. Custardy Peaches and Bananas (see page 144). Glass of diluted fruit juice

Snacks Fresh fruit

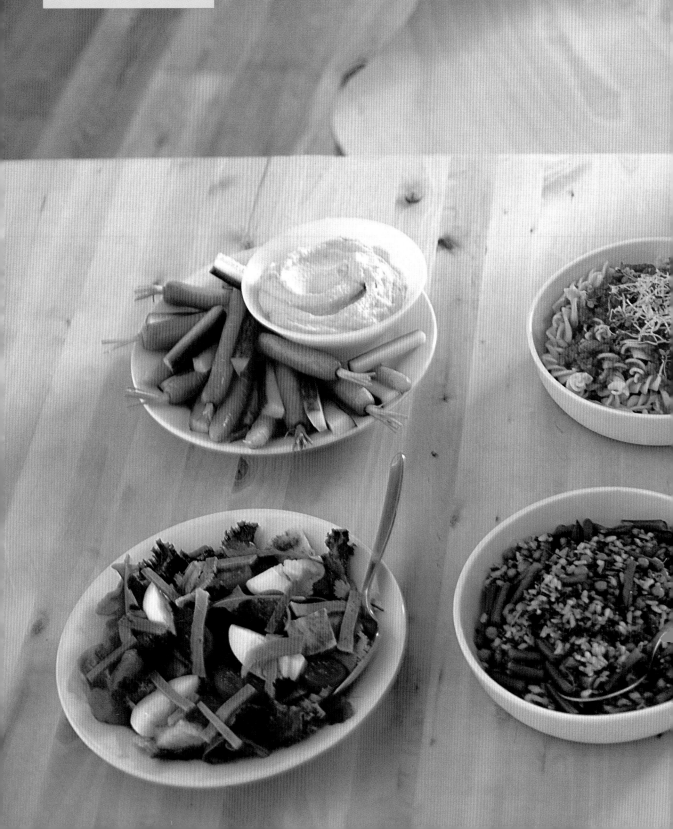

PART 3
Tempting recipes for babies and children

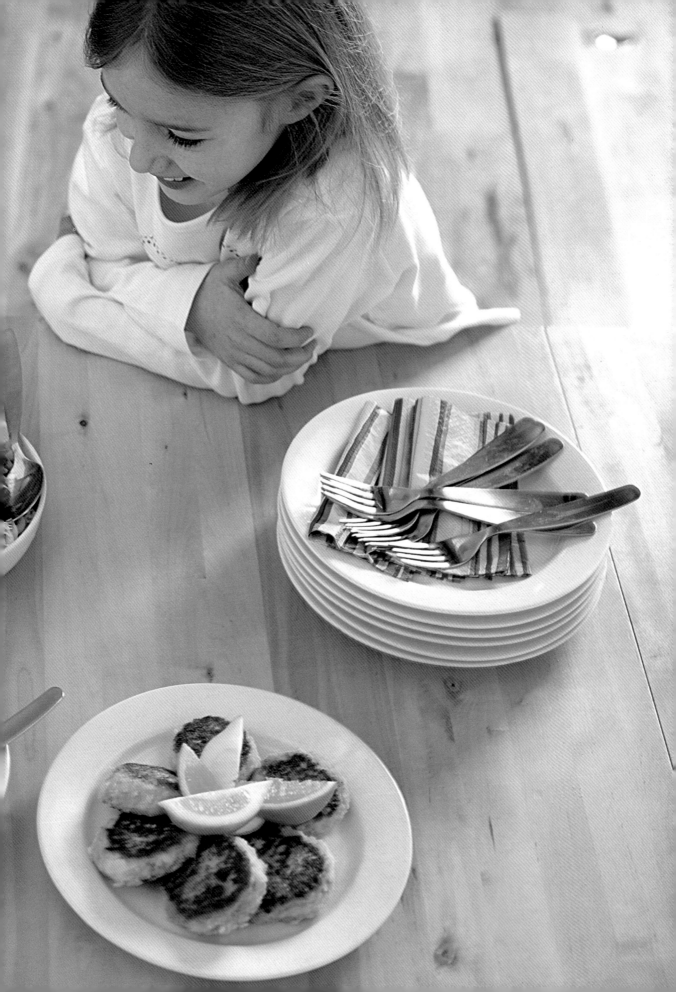

First foods

The age at which you wean from breast to bottle will vary from child to child (see When and why to wean, pages 80–81), because some children grow faster than others and demand more than just their milk at an early stage. The chart given under Meal planners for birth to six months (see pages 84–5) shows examples of when to introduce first purées with bottle feeds during the day.

First foods

■ Fruits: choose from cooked and puréed apple or pear for the first two weeks. Follow with apricot and peach, then melon (all types), nectarine, papaya, kiwi, prune, banana, plum, mango, cherry, raspberry and avocado.

■ Vegetables: sweet potato, courgette, cauliflower, broccoli, carrots, parsnips, leeks, celery, peas, spinach, tomato, sweet peppers (red and yellow), pumpkin and butternut squash.

■ Grains and pulses: brown rice (or baby rice), millet, oats, barley, quinoa, wheat (but not before nine months old), polenta (maize), semolina, lentils, butter beans, flageolet beans and split peas.

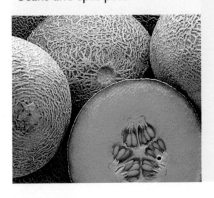

Purées

The first foods to be introduced should have the consistency of a semi-liquid purée, ensuring that all the lumps and bumps have been well smoothed out. New foods should be introduced one at a time, three to four days apart, in order to identify any possible intolerances (rashes, a flushed face or itchy dry patches on the arms and legs). Remember to allow your baby to smell the food as well as taste it – the whole experience is a new one and may take some getting used to. First foods should be mild in flavour and easy to digest – see the list (left) for recommended foods. All meals should be prepared fresh, but bulk quantities can be made once you have determined that your baby enjoys the taste.

Each recipe serves four portions, or two larger portions for older babies

First fruit and vegetable purées

Pear Purée (or other single fruit)

2 medium ripe pears
2 tablespoons water

■ Peel and chop the pears roughly, taking care to remove all the pips.
■ Place in a heavy-bottomed saucepan with the water and simmer gently until the fruit has softened to a purée and absorbed most or all of the water (about 10 minutes).
■ Purée finely and allow to cool before serving.

Carrot Purée (or other single vegetable)

2 medium carrots
3–4 tablespoons water

- Thoroughly wash and peel the carrots, cutting off the tops and tails.
- Chop the carrots finely and add them to the water in a heavy-bottomed pan. Cook over a gentle heat for 15 minutes or until soft.
- Purée finely and allow to cool before serving.

Three-Fruit Purée

2 dried apricots (soaked in water overnight)
1 medium apple
1 peach
2 tablespoons water

- Retain the apricot-soaking water to cook the apple in.
- Wash, peel and core the apple, then simmer gently in the apricot water to a soft consistency (10–12 minutes).
- Score the peach in quarters, then submerge in boiling water for 1–2 minutes to soften the skin; remove the skin with a paring knife.
- Purée all the fruits together, adding more water as necessary to reach the desired consistency. Allow to cool before serving.

Three-Vegetable Purée

1 medium potato
6 tablespoons water
225 g (8 oz) broccoli florets
225 g (8 oz) baby spinach

- Peel the potato and dice finely.
- Place in a pan with the water and simmer gently for 5 minutes.
- Place the broccoli florets in a steamer over the potatoes, and continue cooking for a further 10 minutes, adding the washed spinach to the steamer after the first 5 minutes.
- Purée all the vegetables together to a creamy consistency, and allow to cool before serving.

Other fruit-purée combinations

- Apple, pear and nectarine
- Banana and apricot (the banana needs no cooking)
- Peach, apple and raspberry (the peach and raspberry need no cooking)
- Avocado and pear (the avocado needs no cooking)
- Mango and banana
- Plum and pear

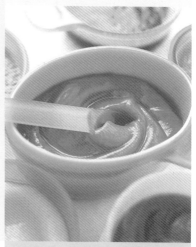

Other vegetable-purée combinations

- Butternut squash and leek
- Cauliflower and parsnip
- Potato, pea and broccoli
- Sweet potato and red pepper
- Tomato, carrot and squash

Ice cube purées

Once you know that your child likes a particular type of purée you can make a batch and freeze it in individual blocks in an ice cube tray.

First grain/pulse purées

Brown Rice Purée

175 g (6 oz) brown rice
900 ml water

The taste is naturally sweet, and offers a more nutrient-rich purée than the ready-made baby-rice alternative.

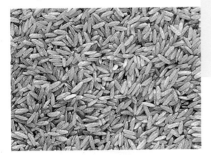

- Simmer the rice gently (with no added salt) in the water, until very soft (about 30–40 minutes).
- Purée finely to a creamy consistency. Allow to cool before serving.

Quinoa Purée

175 g (6 oz) quinoa
600 ml (1 pt) water
1 peach, peeled and chopped (optional)

Quinoa (pronounced 'keenwa') has one of the highest protein ratios of any grain and is therefore ideal for the vegetarian baby. This is an ancient grain, which has not been cloned or tampered with and is virtually tasteless, thus allowing fruits or vegetables to be added to suit your baby's taste.

- Place the quinoa in a heavy-bottomed pan, cover with a lid and simmer gently in the water for 10 minutes.
- Remove from the heat and allow to stand for a further 15 minutes, until most of the water has been absorbed and the grain has fluffed up to a full round-ball consistency.
- Purée to a smooth consistency, adding either cooked vegetables or fruit (such as the peach) to taste. Allow to cool before serving.

Lentil Purée

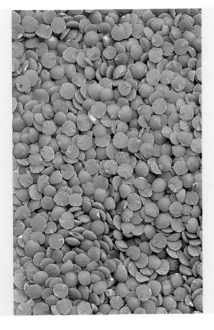

1 small sweet potato
600 ml (1 pt) water
1 medium leek
100 g (4 oz) red lentils

- Peel and finely chop the sweet potato, then place in a heavy-bottomed pan with the water.
- Thoroughly wash and finely chop the leek, then add it to the pan with the lentils.
- Simmer for 25 minutes until the lentils are soft. Purée all the ingredients until smooth, and allow to cool before serving.

First meat and fish purées

White Fish and Vegetable Purée

1 medium carrot, washed and peeled
1 medium red pepper, cored and deseeded
100 g (4 oz) potato (white or sweet), peeled
135 g (5 oz) plaice or cod fillet, skin removed
85 ml (3 fl oz) milk or water
1 bay leaf (optional)

- Chop all the vegetables, then place in a pan with enough water to cover them.
- Cover with a lid and simmer for about 20 minutes until tender, then purée coarsely.
- Place the fish in a separate pan with the milk or water and the bay leaf, if desired (for added flavour).
- Simmer gently for 5–7 minutes until the fish is cooked and flakes easily. Check carefully for bones and remove any that are found.
- Add the fish and liquid to the vegetable mixture and mash with a fork or purée to the desired consistency. Serve the purée warm.

Chicken and white fish are the best sources of animal protein to add to first purées, since both have a relatively bland taste that is likely to appeal to your baby. However, do not introduce either of these before the age of four months.

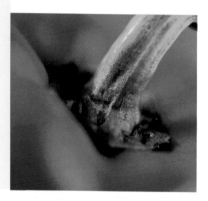

Chicken, Squash and Courgette Purée

75 g (3 oz) chicken breast
50 g (2 oz) leeks, washed
50 g (2 oz) butternut squash, peeled
1 medium courgette, peeled
600 ml (1 pt) water
fresh herbs to taste (thyme or tarragon)

- Wash the chicken and chop the vegetables.
- Place them in a saucepan with the water and herbs, and simmer gently for 20–25 minutes until all the vegetables are soft and the chicken is cooked through.
- Purée roughly and cool to the desired temperature.

Squashes are rich in beta-carotene, an important anti-oxidant required to support your child's immune system.

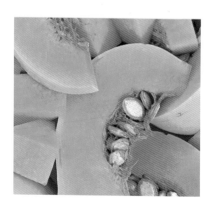

First cereals

and breakfast must-haves

Making the move from breast and bottle to first purées is the first step in weaning, but the transition to cereals (other than baby rice) is just as important. Cereals contain a high ratio of B vitamins, which are essential for growth and energy, so understanding how and when to use them allows you to give your child the very best in early nutrition.

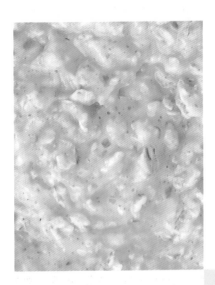

From an early age, your child will have enjoyed the natural sugars found in many fruit and vegetable purées, and it is therefore important to continue to provide a measure of that natural sweetness in cereal-based breakfasts, otherwise children may find these rather dull to the palate. Commercial cereals are predominantly made from refined wheat products, and offer little in the way of sustenance over an extended period of time, so your child is likely to feel more hungry when eating these types of cereals. Having a good range of different grains and flakes in the larder (see The storage cupboard, pages 46–7) will make breakfasts interesting and varied.

These recipes all serve four portions for under 7 and two to three portions for the older age-groups.

First cereals

Oaty Fruity Porridge

100 g (4 oz) oats
300 ml (10 fl oz) apple juice
300 ml (10 fl oz) milk, Vanilla Rice Dream or Oatly (milk alternatives)
2 fresh apricots, or 2 dried apricots soaked overnight, chopped
1 medium apple, cored and diced
1 tablespoon raisins or sultanas
½–1 banana (optional extra, for puréed version only)

- Soak the oats overnight in the apple juice to allow the sweetness of the grain to emerge. Store in the fridge overnight.
- Place the oats in a pan with the milk, or milk alternative, and heat gently for about 10 minutes.
- Add the fruits, then either purée the porridge or serve warm, as it is.

Note: if preparing this dish for babies under one year old, all the fruits should be cooked lightly in half a pint (500 ml) apple juice and milk; otherwise, they may be chopped to similar sizes and added to the porridge when it has been made.

Brainy Seed Granola Cereal

1 teaspoon sunflower seeds
1 teaspoon pumpkin seeds
1 teaspoon sesame seeds
1 teaspoon linseeds
50 g (2 oz) millet (or barley) flakes
50 g (2 oz) oat flakes
1 tablespoon good-quality honey (preferably organic)

- Preheat the oven to 175°C/350°F/Gas Mark 4.
- Grind all the seeds roughly together in a coffee grinder or food processor, then set aside.
- Place the millet (or barley) and oat flakes on a flat baking tray and drizzle the honey all over them. Place in the hot oven for 10 minutes, until the honey has melted and spread.
- Remove the tray from the oven, mix the flakes with a wooden spoon to coat them thoroughly with the honey, then return to the oven for a further 10 minutes.
- Remove from the oven and stir in the seed mix. Spread it flat on the baking tray and allow to cool.
- Scrape off the cereal, then break it up to create smaller pieces. Keep in an airtight container until required.
- Serve with fresh fruit and milk, or milk alternative.

Note: this recipe also makes a healthy granola bar, or granola bites. Simply draw the mixture together when the cooking time has finished, add the seed mix, combine thoroughly, and then roll the mixture into granola bars or balls, for healthy snacking. (Doubling the quantities will allow you to make both the cereal and the snack at the same time.)

Breakfast must-haves

Rice and Fruit Compote

150g (5 oz) brown rice
100g (4 oz) apple (or pear) juice
85 ml (3 fl oz) water
2 medium pears, peeled
50 g (2 oz) berries, such as raspberries or blueberries
85 ml (3 fl oz) milk, Vanilla Rice Dream or Oatly (milk alternatives)

- Soak the rice overnight in half the apple juice and the water, to allow it to swell (this saves on cooking time). Store in the fridge overnight.
- Chop the pears roughly and mix with the berries of your choice.
- Cook the rice in the remaining apple juice and the milk, or milk alternative, until creamy and soft in consistency.
- Beat in the fruits and heat through for 1–2 minutes. Serve warm.

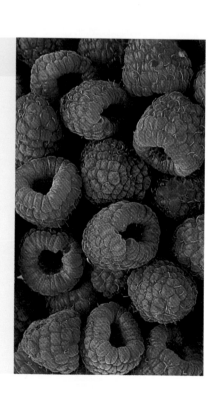

Buckwheat Pancakes

Note: these pancakes store well if they are frozen. Place a piece of kitchen paper between each pancake, to prevent sticking and breaking when defrosting, and then store in a freezer bag.

1 egg
120 ml (4 fl oz) milk, Rice Dream or Oatly (milk alternatives)
100 g (4 oz) buckwheat flour

- Whisk the egg with the milk, or milk alternative, then add the flour, until a light, fluffy batter has been created. Allow to stand for 10 minutes. (Alternatively, this mixture may be made the night before and stored overnight in the fridge).
- Drop small ladles of batter into the centre of a non-stick pan, then swirl the pan around to allow the formation of wafer-thin pancakes (this requires a bit of practice!).
- Turn the pancake over after 1 minute and allow it to cook on the other side, then remove it from the pan and place on a plate.
- Continue the process until all the batter has been used up.

Fluffy Scrambled Eggs

1 egg per child
½ teaspoon light olive oil
1 tablespoon milk, Rice Dream or Oatly (milk alternatives)

- Whisk all the ingredients together, then pour into a pan that has been heated over a medium heat for 1–2 minutes.
- Stir continuously for 3–4 minutes, until the desired consistency is attained. Serve with Buckwheat Pancakes (see above).

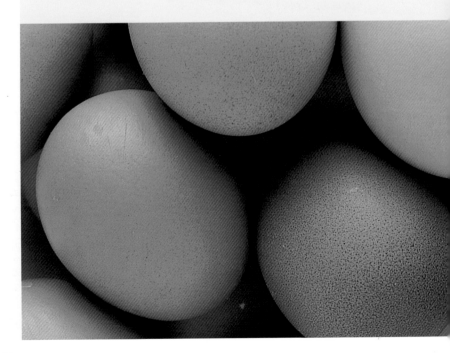

Essential main meals

Main meals can be given to children for lunches, teas or suppers, depending on age and the regularity with which you need to feed your child. Meat, poultry, fish and vegetable dishes are included in this section, and may be combined to form a larger meal or part of a family meal. Some of the vegetable dishes are perfect for light suppers or teas when your child is not feeling very hungry, or for giving close to bedtime, when a heavier meal is unsuitable.

**All recipes serve four medium portions
(or six portions for children of a very young age).**

Chicken and Lentil Soup

1 leftover chicken carcase
2 carrots, chopped
1 parsnip, chopped
1 medium onion, chopped
1 stick of celery, chopped
1 clove garlic (optional), chopped
2 tablespoons Puy or red lentils (double the quantity if omitting the chicken)
black pepper
pinch of dried thyme/sprig of fresh thyme
1 large chicken breast (about 150 g/5 oz), chopped
60 g (2¼ oz) frozen peas

- Place the chicken carcase, together with the carrots, parsnip, onion, celery, garlic (if desired), lentils, black pepper and thyme into a large pan, and cover with water.
- Bring to the boil, then reduce to a simmer for 45 minutes. Make sure that the liquid does not boil continuously, as this will overcook the vegetables.
- Remove the chicken carcase and any remaining small bones. Add the chopped meat to the pan and add the peas.
- Heat the mixture thoroughly, then serve the soup in deep bowls to prevent spilling. (Alternatively, remove the carcase and all bones, then add the chicken breast and peas, heat through and blend the ingredients to create a smooth soup.)

Although soup tends to appeal to the older child, a 'meal-in-a-bowl' is also tempting for younger children and allows you to add extra vegetables where you might not otherwise be able to persuade your child to eat them. This recipe allows for enormous variety, as you can substitute the specified vegetables for other root vegetables in season, or for any particular vegetables that your child has a liking for. For vegetarians, the chicken may be omitted.

Note: if you are making a vegetarian soup with just the lentils, increase the amount of seasoning, and add 1 tablespoon of vegetable bouillon stock powder to increase the soup's flavour.

Bean Pot

Beans are an excellent vegetarian source of protein, and they provide plenty of energy and warmth throughout the winter months. However, do not introduce beans prior to the age of six months, because your child will not have sufficient digestive enzymes to cope with them. The aim of this dish is to create an interest in your child in all the different colours and textures. All the vegetables should be chopped into different sizes, so that children can identify which vegetable is which.

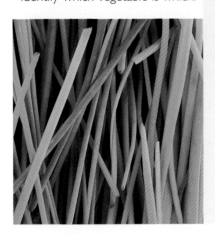

2 tablespoons olive oil
1 medium onion, peeled and finely diced
½ medium butternut squash, peeled and diced
5 cm (2 in) strip of kombu (optional) (a Japanese dried seaweed that reduces the wind caused by beans and pulses)
1 red pepper, cored, deseeded and chopped into small strips
1 yellow pepper, cored, deseeded and chopped into small strips
50 g (2 oz) French beans, with the ends removed
1 x 50g g (2 oz) tin of sweetcorn
1.2 litres (2 pt) water
1 tablespoon of good-quality vegetable stock powder
1 x 225 g (8 oz) tin butter, kidney or haricot beans, rinsed
50 g (2 oz) crème fraîche (optional)

- Heat the olive oil gently in a large heavy-based pan.
- Add the onion and butternut squash, and gently sauté until the onions are transparent.
- Add the kombu (if desired) and all the remaining vegetables except for the butter, kidney or haricot beans, and toss in the oil for 2–3 minutes.
- Boil the water separately, then add to the vegetables, stirring in the vegetable stock and the beans of your choice. Cover and simmer gently for 25–30 minutes, until the vegetables are still firm, but not hard.
- Either serve the dish as it is, with chunks of good wholemeal or rye bread, or purée it and serve as a creamy soup, adding the crème fraîche at the last minute.

Beany-Burgers (or Beany Balls)

These delicious bean-balls or bean-burgers should not be reserved purely for the vegetarian child – they are ideal for picnic lunches, lunch boxes or as an easy alternative to the hamburger. Beans and pulses are a rich source of protein essential for growth and repair, and the wide variety of beans available should cater for different tastes. This dish is not suitable for children under nine months.

1 x 350 g (12 oz) tin flageolet, kidney or haricot beans
350 g (12 oz) potato, sweet potato, carrots or butternut squash (or a combination of any of these), peeled and roughly chopped
2 tablespoons olive oil
1 onion, finely chopped
1 tablespoon tomato purée or passata
1 tablespoon plain flour (to bind the mixture); chickpea or gram flour may be used for children on a wheat-free diet
1 large tomato, to garnish

- Put the beans in a sieve and rinse thoroughly under running water. Allow to stand for several minutes to drain off all the liquid, then place them in a large bowl and mash with a fork. Put to one side.

- Meanwhile, simmer the potato, sweet potato, carrots or squash in a little water until tender, then drain and mash.
- Heat half the olive oil in a separate pan, and gently sauté the onion until transparent.
- Combine the onions and mashed vegetables with the bean mixture and stir thoroughly, adding the tomato purée or passata.
- Add the flour to bind all the ingredients together, and shape into four medium Beany-Burgers or 10–12 Beany Balls.
- Heat the remaining olive oil and fry the shapes gently until lightly golden (not burnt) and completely heated through.
- The Beany-Burgers may be served with toasted pitta pockets, rye bread or muffins, and sliced tomatoes for garnish. Alternatively, the Beany Balls may be served with rice and Honeyed Vegetable Stir-Fry (see page 140).

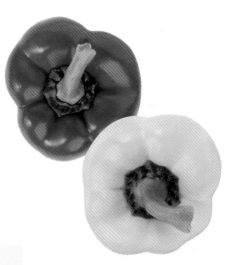

Mixed Vegetable Mash

100 g (4 oz) Maris Piper or other mashing potatoes, peeled and chopped
1 tablespoon vegetable bouillon stock powder
100 g (4 oz) swede (or other root vegetable), butternut squash, broccoli, courgettes or carrots, peeled and chopped
25 g (1 oz) butter or olive oil
black pepper
85 ml (3 fl oz) milk, Rice Dream or Oatly (milk alternatives)

- Place the potatoes in sufficient water to cover them, adding the stock powder to enhance their flavour.
- Bring to the boil and cook for 10 minutes, before adding the swede or other root vegetables (or 15 minutes before adding the squash, broccoli, courgettes, carrots or other softer vegetables).
- Simmer until all the vegetables are soft. Strain, reserving about 2 tablespoons of stock, then return the vegetables to the pan.
- Add the butter or olive oil and a little ground black pepper.
- Mash thoroughly, then add the milk, or milk substitute, until the mixture is creamy-smooth. If the mixture is too firm, add one or two tablespoons of the stock reserved from boiling the vegetables.
- Serve with any main dish, or top with grated cheese.

It's amazing how many children will eat mashed vegetables, although they won't even look at whole ones! To save time when preparing a selection of vegetables, choose potato as your base, then another one or two vegetables of a different colour; you can add these to the boiling potatoes near the end of the cooking, then blend them all together.

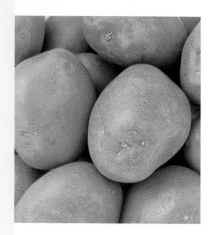

This sweetened vegetable dish is an excellent way to tempt children to experiment with a selection of vegetables. The combination of soy sauce and honey is taken from Indonesia and China. Take care not to add more honey than is recommended in the recipe. Good-quality honey has natural anti-bacterial properties, so this is an excellent dish to give your child when he has a cold or is a little run-down. To make this into a main dish, you could chop up and add a grilled or baked chicken breast after the vegetables have been cooked, but before the soy sauce and honey are added.

Honeyed Vegetable Stir-Fry

2 tablespoons light olive oil
1 clove garlic, finely chopped
1 small onion, peeled and chopped
1 cm (½ in) of fresh ginger root, peeled and finely chopped (optional)
1 red pepper, cored, deseeded and cut into strips
1 green pepper, cored, deseeded and cut into strips
175 g (6 oz) baby corn, sliced in half lengthways
175 g (6 oz) mangetout or snap-peas, washed and trimmed
50 g (2 oz) fresh or frozen peas
1 tablespoon soy sauce or tamari (wheat-free soy sauce)
1 tablespoon good-quality honey

- Heat the olive oil in a heavy-based pan and add the garlic, onion and ginger (if desired), tossing the mixture continuously for 2–3 minutes.
- Add the peppers, baby corn and mangetout or snap-peas, and continue cooking for another 2 minutes.
- Add the fresh or frozen peas, heat through and then drizzle soy sauce or tamari over all the vegetables.
- Stir in the honey to lightly coat the mixture. Serve immediately.

Pasta Bows with Ham and Peas

350–400 g (12–14 oz) wholewheat, corn or buckwheat pasta bows
  (use shapes for younger children)
2 tablespoons corn or olive oil
4 large slices of honey-roast or other ham, chopped
50 g (2 oz) fresh or frozen peas or sweetcorn
4 tablespoons tomato passata or red pesto sauce

- Cook the pasta in sufficient water to cover it amply, adding 1 tablespoon corn or olive oil to prevent sticking. Simmer for 10–12 minutes until firm, but not mushy. Drain and set aside.
- Heat the remaining oil gently in a pan and sauté the chopped ham and the peas or sweetcorn for 2 minutes.
- Add the passata or pesto sauce, and cook for a further 1–2 minutes to combine the flavours, stirring the sauce into the pasta to coat it thoroughly. Serve immediately.

There is no getting away from the popularity of pasta, and the ease and speed with which it is prepared makes it an inevitable regular at the kitchen table. To avoid overloading your child with the wheat from pasta and other standbys (bread, biscuits and cakes), try using corn pasta or buckwheat macaroni (despite its name, buckwheat actually comes from the rhubarb family) as alternatives. These both require a little oil added to the boiling water, to reduce the stickiness of their texture.

Note: for a vegetarian option, use 100 g (4 oz) red kidney beans or borlotti beans instead of the ham.

Fisherman's Pasta Bake

350 g (12 oz) wholewheat or corn macaroni
1 tablespoon sunflower oil
225 g (8 oz) fresh fish fillets, deboned and skinned (or 225 g/8 oz tinned
*   fish of your choice, with the bones removed)*
1 carrot, finely chopped
1 tablespoon vegetable bouillon stock powder
25 g (1 oz) butter or Vitaquell (non-hydrogenated butter alternative)
25 g (1 oz) plain flour or cornflour (to thicken the sauce)
175 ml (6 fl oz) milk, Rice Dream or Oatly (milk alternatives)
black pepper

- Cook the macaroni in a deep pan, in sufficient water to cover it amply, adding the sunflower oil to prevent sticking. Simmer for about 10–12 minutes or until the pasta is still firm, but 'gives' to the fork.

- Meanwhile, poach the fish fillets and carrots in water with the stock powder, in a shallow uncovered pan, over a medium heat for 10–15 minutes. Remove the fish and flake it on a dish, then set aside. Retain the water from the poached fish to add to the sauce.

- Melt the butter or Vitaquell gently in a separate pan, and make a roux by adding the flour or cornflour to form a paste. Cook over a medium heat for 2–3 minutes, then add the milk, or milk alternative, a little at a time and stirring continuously, to create a creamy sauce.

- Add black pepper to taste, and 25–50 ml (1–2 fl oz) of the fish stock to add flavour and keep the sauce smooth and not too thick. Take the pan off the heat.

- Arrange the pasta in a shallow baking dish, placing the fish in and around the whole dish, rather than just on top. Pour over the sauce, making sure that you cover the whole dish.

- Place under the grill for 5–10 minutes to lightly brown the topping, and serve with vegetables of your choice.

If your child is reluctant to eat much fish, then combining it with pasta is an excellent way of making it more palatable. Fish is such an important food for growth, immunity and repair that it should be served at least two or three times a week. Choose from salmon, tuna, trout, plaice or haddock. Make sure you buy fillets that have been thoroughly deboned (or use tinned varieties for a faster meal).

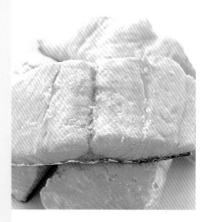

Sticky Lamb Cutlets

Red meat is an important source of iron for children, which is needed on a more regular basis during childhood growth than during adulthood. Lamb is one of most children's favourites and has the advantage of being a low allergen risk. Ideally choose organic or best-quality cutlets, as cheaper cuts do not offer the same nutritional value.

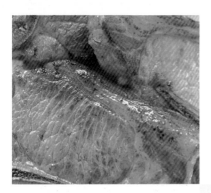

juice of 2 lemons
1 teaspoon soy sauce
1 teaspoon sesame oil (optional, but do not use where there is a risk of nut allergy)
2 teaspoons honey
1 teaspoon tomato purée
black pepper
4 lamb cutlets

■ Mix together the lemon juice, soy sauce, sesame oil (if desired), honey, tomato purée and black pepper, then spread over both sides of the lamb cutlets.
■ Leave the paste to infuse its flavours for at least 1 hour (the paste may be prepared in the morning and left in the fridge until tea or supper).
■ Place the cutlets under a medium-to-high grill for 4–5 minutes on each side.
■ Meanwhile, reduce any remaining marinade in a pan over a high heat for a few minutes, taking care not to burn it.
■ Serve the cutlets and marinade immediately, with mixed vegetable mash, or baked potatoes and broccoli and carrots.

Chicken with Rice

Note: do not leave this dish to stand for more than half an hour after cooking without either eating it or placing it (once cool) in the fridge, because the risk of bacterial infection is far higher when chicken and rice are cooked together.

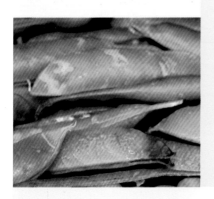

2 medium-sized chicken breasts or 4 legs, skin removed
1 lemon, cut in half
175 g (6 oz) wholegrain (brown) or plain white rice, thoroughly rinsed
2 carrots, chopped
1 medium onion, peeled and chopped
50 g (2 oz) mangetout, French beans or fresh or frozen peas
1 red pepper, cored, deseeded and cut into strips
1.2 litres (2 pt) water
2 tablespoons vegetable bouillon stock powder
black pepper
1 bay leaf, or other herbs of your choice (tarragon, thyme, parsley)
1 tablespoon soy sauce or tamari (wheat-free soy sauce)

■ Wash the chicken and rub it all over with the lemon (this is an Oriental technique to ensure that any bacteria are cleaned from the chicken before cooking).
■ Place the chicken in a deep heavy-based pan and add the rice, spreading it out evenly.

- Add all the vegetables, then pour over the water and stock powder, stirring the mixture to ensure that there is an even distribution of all the ingredients throughout the pan.
- Add the black pepper, herbs and soy sauce or tamari for flavour.
- Cover the pan tightly and cook over a medium heat (once the water has come to the boil) for 35–40 minutes, or until the rice is cooked. When it is ready, the dish should have absorbed all of the water and sit ready for serving straight from the pan.

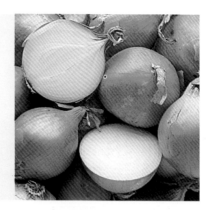

Almost-Adult Beef Curry

1 tablespoon olive oil
1 large onion, peeled and chopped
1 clove garlic, grated or crushed
2 leeks (outer skins removed), chopped into rounds
50 g (2 oz) potatoes, chopped and par-boiled for 10 minutes
2 tablespoons mild curry powder
400–450 g (14–16 oz) lean sirloin or fillet beef, cubed
2 tablespoons tomato purée
300 ml (10 fl oz) vegetable or beef stock
1 teaspoon cornflour
3 tablespoons natural yoghurt (optional)

- Heat the oil in a heavy-based pan over a moderate heat, and sauté the onion and garlic until transparent.
- Add the leeks, potatoes, curry powder and beef, stirring thoroughly to ensure that all the meat and vegetables are coated with the paste.
- Cook for 1–2 minutes, stirring continuously, and then add the tomato purée and stock. Bring to the boil, then simmer for 35–40 minutes.
- Mix one tablespoon of the curry sauce with the cornflour to make a paste, then return the paste to the curry, stirring it in thoroughly. Cook for a further 15 minutes until the curry sauce has thickened to the required consistency.
- Add the yoghurt to cool the curry, if it is too spicy. Serve immediately with rice.

In the Far East, rice is served with almost every meal; indeed, some dishes are one-pot meals, where everything is cooked in one dish, thereby preserving all the nutritional content. Children tend to love rice, as it is naturally slightly sweet, and it provides plenty of the B vitamins required for energy and brain function. This one-pot dish can be adapted to incorporate your children's favourite vegetables.

It is surprising how many children enjoy the flavours of curry, and it offers an excellent way of serving meat with several vegetables in a single dish. Curry is also a good means of using up leftovers, such as new potatoes, beef from the Sunday roast or an excess of root vegetables. Start your child on a mild-flavoured curry to adapt her palate to the taste.

Puddings and treats

It would be easier at mealtimes if all puddings and treats could be served first, and the main courses second: there would never be a fuss about what was being served, because puddings and treats are invariably sweet. However, it is important not to treat this part of the meal as a reward, only to be given if the rest of the meal has been satisfactorily consumed (see Food for reward, pages 60–61), but rather as *part* of the whole meal.

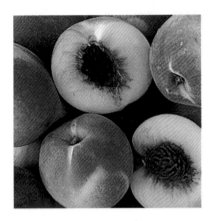

In the following recipes, fruits have been used more often than any other ingredient, since they offer the highest nutritional variety and are often refused in their raw form by all children at certain ages. I like to think that no family kitchen is ever without a tempting bowl of fruit, from which children may take items at any time of the day, rather than being offered a piece of fruit only at the end of a meal. It is far better to allow children, when they are hungry, to help themselves to a piece of fruit, rather than have them looking endlessly for the next piece of chocolate or bag of crisps.

All recipes serve four persons or two adolescents.

Custardy Peaches and Bananas

Custard is highly nutritious, and offers all the benefits of iron, calcium and B vitamins (in the egg yolks), with beta-carotene, vitamin C (in the peaches), and phosphorus and magnesium (in the bananas). Bananas are also a rich source of tryptophan, which helps to encourage sound sleep, so this is an ideal pudding for tea or supper to relax and calm your child. You can replace the peaches and banana with other fruits, depending on the season.

Note: the custard will set into a firm consistency, so it is possible to put the mixture into moulds to be turned out onto the plate, for special occasions.

2 large egg yolks (reserve the whites for meringues)
1 teaspoon cornflour
1 tablespoon clear honey
1 teaspoon vanilla extract (in liquid form)
300 ml (10 fl oz) milk, Vanilla Rice Dream or Oatly (milk alternatives)
2 bananas
2 peaches, peeled

- Whisk the egg yolks, and combine with the cornflour, honey and vanilla extract in a heavy-based pan.
- In a separate pan, warm the milk gently, then add it to the egg mixture, stirring it continuously over a low heat until slightly thickened. (Some children prefer their custard much thicker than others, particularly if you are going to mix it with fruits and place it in the fridge – so try different consistencies until they are satisfied.)
- Slice the bananas and peaches into a serving dish, and pour the custard over the top. Serve either warm, or chilled from the fridge.

Apple Bombs

4 red apples, or Granny Smiths, cored but not peeled
4 teaspoons raisins or sultanas
4 dates, chopped and the stones removed
2 tablespoons clear honey

- Preheat the oven to 180°C/350°F/Gas Mark 4.
- Stuff the apple cavities tightly with a mixture of the dried fruits.
- Put the apples on a buttered baking dish, then drizzle a little honey over each apple cavity, allowing it to drip through the fruits while cooking.
- Place the baking tray in the centre of the oven for 40–50 minutes, until the apples have softened but not fallen apart. Serve with custard or crème fraîche.
- You can use 2 tablespoons blueberries/blackberries as a summer alternative to the dried fruits suggested above.

Most children love apples, either raw or cooked, and they are so easy to place in the oven to bake while you are preparing the remainder of the meal. Adding other fruits to the apple cavities increases the nutritional value of this pudding, but avoid soft berries, as they tend to fall apart. Apples are particularly useful when your child has been unwell, because they help to remove toxins from the digestive tract, and contain plenty of immune-boosting nutrients.

Date and Oat Flapjacks

50 g (2 oz) butter
75 g (3 oz) dark brown (muscovado) sugar
225 g (8 oz) rolled oats (porridge oats)
25 g (1 oz) sultanas or raisins
50 g (2 oz) dates, chopped and the stones removed
25 g (1 oz) dried apricots, chopped
4 tablespoons sunflower or rapeseed oil

- Preheat the oven to 180°C/350°F/Gas Mark 4.
- Line a 30 x 20 cm (12 x 8 in) baking tin with greaseproof or baking paper.
- Mix the butter and sugar in a pan, then melt them together over a low heat until all the sugar has dissolved.
- Add the remaining ingredients, and mix together thoroughly.
- Turn the mixture into the baking tin, and place in the oven for 30 minutes. Remove and allow to cool for 10–15 minutes before slicing. Do not attempt to remove the flapjacks from the tin until they have completely cooled. Keep in an airtight container for up to one week.

There are many versions of this recipe; some may include more fruits, and others nuts. Involve your child in the cooking, as some kids have a tendency to avoid foods of which they are uncertain. Flapjacks are so easy to prepare; you can do a weekly 'make and bake'. Dates, figs and apricots are all excellent sources of iron, as well as beta-carotene, which is important for the immune system, and calcium for building strong bones. Oats are packed with B vitamins for energy, and with zinc, which is required for a healthy digestive and immune system.

Note: these flapjacks should not be served to children under one year old, as the oats are difficult to digest in their wholegrain form and may represent a choking risk.

Carrot-Cake Muffins

These muffins are an ideal way to provide children who do not eat many vegetables with carrots, which are rich in beta-carotene, an essential nutrient for the immune system and for promoting good eyesight. They are also an excellent addition to a lunch box, or as a whole food when children first come home from school.

175 g (6 oz) wholemeal self-raising flour
75 g (3 oz) dark brown (muscovado) sugar
2 teaspoons baking powder
3 eggs
1 teaspoon vanilla extract (in liquid form)
225 g (8 oz) carrots, grated
120 ml (4 fl oz) rapeseed or sunflower oil
small pinch of nutmeg or ground ginger, to flavour

- Preheat the oven to 180°C/350°F/Gas Mark 4.
- Sift the flour into a large mixing bowl, then add the sugar and baking powder.
- Whisk the eggs and add them to the flour mixture, together with the vanilla extract, the grated carrots and the oil and spice flavourings. Mix thoroughly, making sure all the flour has been taken up by the mixture.
- Line a 12 x mini-cake tray with paper cake liners, and spoon the mixture evenly into each one. Bake in the middle of the oven for 25–30 minutes, or until golden brown, but not burned.
- Take the tray out of the oven and remove each cake liner. Place all the muffins on a wire rack to cool. Remove the papers only when the muffins have cooled, to prevent them breaking.
- Serve warm with crème fraîche as a pudding, or cooled as a snack. Keep in an airtight container for up to one week.

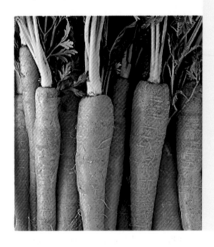

Fruity Rice Pudding

Rice pudding is one of those staples that most children love. It is a perfect dessert to add a lot of fruit to for sweetening (instead of pounds of sugar) and these can be varied to suit the season. Rice pudding is suitable for all ages, and is one of the first foods to give your baby. Rice is rich in all minerals, but the bleached white variety has fewer nutrients, so try baking your rice pudding using a wholegrain brown rice, which simply requires longer cooking.

1 teaspoon butter
100 g (4 oz) wholegrain brown rice (or pudding rice for younger babies and infants)
1.2 litres (2 pt) milk, Vanilla Rice Dream or Oatly (milk alternatives)
½ teaspoon vanilla essence
2 teaspoons caster sugar or honey
4 tablespoons fruit purée (pear, apple, raspberry, cherry or blackberry)

- Preheat the oven to 150°C/300°F/Gas Mark 2.
- Rub the butter all round an ovenproof baking dish.
- Place the remaining ingredients in the dish and combine gently with a wooden spoon.
- Bake for about 40 minutes, then remove the dish to stir the rice once. Place the dish back in the oven for 1 hour more, until set. Serve when slightly cooled.

Fruit Fool Flummery

*50 g (2 oz) raspberries, strawberries or blackberries (fresh when in
season, or frozen during the winter)*
2 pears, peeled and chopped
1 nectarine or peach, peeled and chopped
175 g (6 oz) plain bio yoghurt
2 teaspoons clear honey (optional)

- Blend all the fruits together in a food processor or blender, then
  pour into individual bowls.
- Add 2 tablespoons of yoghurt to each bowl, and swirl with a fork
  to create a marbled pattern.
- Drizzle honey over the centre of each dish, if desired

A flummery was traditionally a pudding to which beaten egg whites had been added, to lighten the dish. However, because uncooked egg whites offer an increased risk of food poisoning, it is advisable to replace them with plain natural yoghurt. This is a great way to use a wide variety of fruits throughout the year and to encourage children to eat more fruit, and they tend to lap it up. Choose their favourite fruit as the dominant flavour.

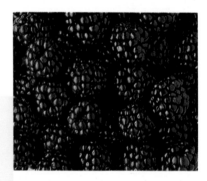

Home-Made Ice-Lollies

450 g (1 lb) fruit (fresh, frozen or rehydrated)
100 g (4 oz) caster sugar
120 ml (4 fl oz) water
25 ml (1 fl oz) apple or orange juice

- Start by blending the fruit to remove any lumps.
- Place the sugar and water in a heavy-based pan and dissolve the
  sugar, until the liquid thickens to a syrup.
- Combine the syrup with the puréed fruit and apple or orange juice,
  and pour into ice-lolly moulds.
- Place in the freezer until fully frozen (at least 4 hours).

Ice-lolly moulds are now widely available at supermarkets, allowing you and your children to make your own ice-lollies. The benefit is that you can regulate the amount of sugar (usually absurdly high in commercial lollies). Use fresh fruits in the summer, and frozen or rehydrated dried fruits in the winter (rehydrate dried apricots by soaking them overnight in warm water – they will treble in size and plumpness). While ice-lollies are not the healthiest of puddings, they are a vast improvement on shop-bought varieties.

Easy alternatives

In an ideal world we would all like to be able to offer our children the very best of fresh foods all the time, but this can be enormously time-consuming and really isn't the only option. Provided you have a well-stocked larder (see The storage cupboard, pages 46–7), you need never be caught without some sort of dish that you can knock together quickly and easily.

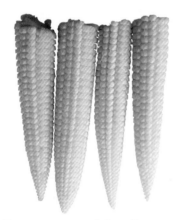

There are several fresh foods that help to complement any larder, including eggs, cheese, milk or a non-dairy alternative (for 'whole-meal-in-a-glass' milkshakes), wholemeal pitta bread (a healthier option for a range of sandwiches) and quick-fix polenta (or maize/corn meal) for healthy pizza bases. Here are some healthy and quickly prepared snack and light-meal options.

All recipes serve four or two larger children (7 plus).

Best vegetables for dipping

- Carrots
- Celery
- Red and green peppers
- Radishes
- Courgettes
- Baby sweetcorn
- Baby tomatoes
- Snap-peas
- French beans
- Small broccoli and cauliflower florets

Whizzies and sticks

Whizzies are dips that have been whizzed up in seconds, served with crudités, or sliced raw vegetables. The latter need not be considered purely an adult snack – young children often cut their teeth (or gums!) on carrot sticks and are drawn to their natural sweetness. Raw vegetable sticks and a variety of easy-to-conjure vegetable and bean dips make an excellent, healthy alternative to packet crisps and other fried commercial snacks.

To save time, prepare enough crudités for several snacking sessions, either between meals to keep blood-sugar levels balanced (for more information on blood-sugar management, see pages 38–41) or as an ideal lunch-box extra.

Ensure that you have good supplies of canned beans and pulses in your store cupboard, as these provide a readily available source of vegetable-based protein for the dips, which in turn will give your child a much richer source of nutrients and energy than sweet treats or packet snacks.

Red Pepper and Butterbean Whizzie

3 red peppers, cored and deseeded
1 x 175 g (6 oz) tin of butterbeans, drained
large pinch of paprika
1 tablespoon crème fraîche, natural yoghurt or soya yoghurt
2 teaspoons olive oil

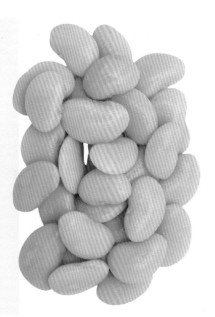

- Combine all the ingredients in a blender or food processor until smooth, adding the oil slowly to reach the desired consistency.
- This whizzie can be kept fresh for up to 3 days, if covered and refrigerated. For lunch boxes and travelling, exclude the crème fraîche or yoghurt, and add more olive oil if necessary, to prevent the dip turning rancid.

Chickpea and Green Pesto Whizzie

1 x 175 g (6 oz) jar of basil or rocket pesto sauce
1 x 175 g (6 oz) tin of chickpeas, drained
freshly ground pepper
lemon juice or cider vinegar to taste

- Combine all the ingredients thoroughly in a blender or food processor, adding the lemon juice or cider vinegar as necessary to reduce the thickness and cut the garlic levels in the pesto to the desired strength.
- This whizzie will probably be best kept for only two or three days, as the ingredients are more likely to ferment than the previous two.

Note: this combination should not be given to children under the age of nine months, as the chickpeas may cause colic or flatulence.

Kidney Bean, Tomato and Mustard Whizzie

1 x 175 g (6 oz) tin red kidney beans
120 ml (4 fl oz) tomato purée or passata (strained tomato sauce)
1 teaspoon wholegrain mustard
1–2 teaspoons water

- Combine all the ingredients except the water in a blender or food processor until smooth, adding the water only if the consistency is too thick.
- This whizzie can be kept fresh for up to 3 days, if covered and refrigerated.

Note: wholegrain mustard is stimulating to the digestive and immune systems, and is excellent added to soups, stews and dips, such as this one. However, if your child develops diarrhoea, it may be that the mustard is too stimulating, in which case reduce the amount by half.

Orzo with Creamy Mushroom Salsa

Orzo is an excellent alternative to wheat-based pasta, as it is made from barley and provides a generous allowance of B vitamins for energy, as well as potassium and magnesium, which contribute towards calming your child! When children crave pasta on an almost daily basis, it usually indicates that they are going through a growth spurt or require 'quick-fix' energy. The mushrooms recommended in this dish have immune-enhancing properties and are not strongly flavoured.

600 ml (1 pt) water for boiling
175 g (6 oz) orzo shapes (from Italian delicatessens or larger supermarkets)

For the sauce
1 small onion, finely sliced
1 tablespoon olive oil
1 x 100 g (4 oz) sliced button mushrooms (fresh or tinned) or 100 g (4 oz) shiitake mushrooms
75 g (3 oz) crème fraîche, plain yoghurt or soya yoghurt
50 g (2 oz) Parmesan cheese (optional)

- Bring the water to the boil in a large pan, then simmer the orzo shapes for 5–10 minutes.
- Drain immediately and do not allow them to stand in the water or they will become soggy. Set aside in a warmed dish or cover the pan with a lid.
- In a separate pan, lightly sauté the onion in the olive oil until transparent, then add the mushrooms, stirring continuously to prevent overcooking, and sauté for another 3–5 minutes.
- Place the onions, mushrooms and crème fraîche or yoghurt in a blender or food processor, and blend until smooth.
- Mix the sauce into the orzo and serve it in bowls, with grated Parmesan, if desired.

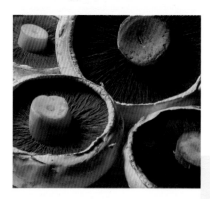

Tuna Tagliatelle

Using fish as a base for a pasta sauce is one the easiest ways to persuade children to eat fish. Fish is a vital ingredient for your child's health, as it is a rich source of essential fats for brain development, soft healthy skin and hormone development. Wholemeal tagliatelle is the preferred option in this dish, as it provides a better source of B vitamins than its white-pasta alternative. Adding broccoli gives this meal an extra nutrient bonus, without placing too much attention on vegetables.

600 ml (1 pt) water for boiling
175 g (6 oz) dried or fresh tagliatelle
1 x 200 g (7 oz) tin tuna in brine, drained
1 x 175 g (6 oz) tin chopped tomatoes, with basil or other herbs
100 g (4 oz) broccoli, chopped
50 g (2 oz) Parmesan cheese (optional)

- Bring the water to the boil in a large pan, then simmer the tagliatelle for 5–6 minutes if dried, or 4–5 minutes if fresh, until al dente. Drain and return to the pan to keep warm.
- Flake the tuna, then place it in a separate pan with the chopped tomatoes and broccoli, mixing them thoroughly.
- Heat the sauce over a moderate heat for 4–5 minutes, then mix it thoroughly into the tagliatelle.
- Serve the tagliatelle in bowls, with grated Parmesan, if desired.

Polenta Pizzas

Makes four medium-sized pizzas or 36 mini ones.

For the base

250 ml (8 fl oz) water
2 teaspoons olive oil
pinch of salt
225 g (8 oz) polenta (quick-mix variety)

- Preheat the oven to 200°C/400°F/Gas Mark 6.
- Bring the water to a simmer in a heavy-based pan with the oil and salt, then pour in the polenta in a steady stream, stirring continuously until it has thickened (the mixture should have the consistency of thick porridge, with no lumps!).
- Turn the mixture out onto a flat baking tray, and place in the oven for 10 minutes until the top has crusted without browning.
- Cut into squares or mini-rectangles, and add a suitable topping (see right) over a generous layer of tomato purée.
- Place under the grill for 5 minutes until the top is gently bubbling. Serve while still warm, or allow to cool and then serve.

Suggested pizza toppings

- Mozzarella cheese
- Mature cheddar
- Chopped red and green peppers
- Halved baby tomatoes
- Sliced mushrooms
- Tinned tuna or salmon
- Sliced, diced ham
- Shredded turkey or chicken breast
- Sliced salami or pre-cooked organic sausages

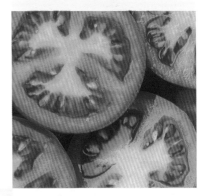

Beany Eggs on Rye

6 eggs
150 ml (5 fl oz) milk (whole milk, not semi-skimmed), Rice Dream or Oatly (milk alternatives)
1 x 175 g (6 oz) tin baked beans
4 pieces sliced rye bread, toasted
50 g (2 oz) baby tomatoes (yellow and red, if available)

- Whisk the eggs and milk together until frothy, then pour into a heavy-based frying pan.
- Scramble the mixture quickly over a moderate heat, then add the baked beans.
- Place the pan under a hot grill for 2–3 minutes, until the eggs have risen and fluffed up on top.
- Divide the dish into four portions and serve it on rye toast, with chopped baby tomatoes on the side.

Rye bread is a good alternative to wheat, having more iron and magnesium – two minerals that are often lacking in a diet that is low on vegetables. Both minerals are important for a strong heart and cardiovascular development.

Eggs are easy to prepare, and provide a wide range of minerals and a good source of sustaining protein. This dish makes a substantial but light tea or supper dish for hungry, tired children. Adding beans or pulses to an egg dish gives it more weight and makes for a more substantial meal.

Vitamin and mineral requirements

The recommended quantity of each nutrient listed below is the *minimum* amount recommended to prevent deficiency of that nutrient at the given ages. It does not recommend *optimum* levels, as this will vary from one child to the next. It is unlikely that your child would consume an excess of any one nutrient within a day, unless you were feeding him on a mono-diet, which is never recommended (unless for allergy testing under supervision by a medical practitioner or nutritionist).

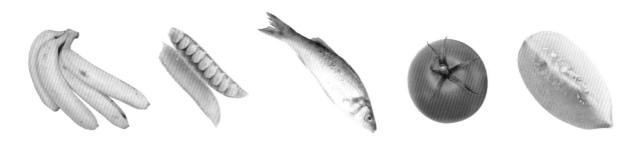

FAT SOLUBLE VITAMINS
Measured in micrograms (mcg) or International Units (IU)

Vitamin A/Beta-Carotene
Required for: Growth, healthy skin and teeth, protects against infection, also an antioxidant and immune booster.

Low levels may cause: Mouth ulcers, dry skin, poor hair condition, night blindness, infections, impaired growth

Required daily doses:

Birth–12 months:	350 mcg
1–3 years:	400 mcg
4–7 years:	500 mcg
8 years–puberty:	700–1000 mcg

Best sources: Canteloupe melons, pumpkin, carrots, peaches, apricots, red peppers, tomatoes, liver, egg yolk, dairy produce, herrings and mackerel

Vitamin D
Required for: Maintaining strong healthy bones by retaining calcium, helps tooth formation and muscle function. Also works with Vitamins A and C to boost immunity and prevent colds. Manufactured in the presence of sunlight.

Low levels may cause: Bone and tooth problems, rickets in extreme cases.

Required daily doses:

Birth–12 months:	8.5 mcg/300 IUs
1–3 years:	7 mcg/250 IUs
4–7 years:	10 mcg/400 IUs (providing exposed to the sunlight)
8 years–puberty:	10 mcg/400 IUs

Best sources: Sardines, herrings, salmon, tuna, dairy produce and egg yolks.

Vitamin E
Required for: Skin health, immune system development, heart and cardiovascular health (it thins the blood). Helps prevent scarring from scratches, grazes and even major surgery.

Low levels may cause: Dry skin, poor wound healing, cracked heels, frequent infections.

Required daily doses:

Birth–12 months:	300–400 IUs
1–3 years:	600 IUs
4–7 years:	700 IUs
8 years to puberty:	800–1000 IUs
Best food sources:	All vegetable oils, avocados, broccoli, almonds, sunflower seeds, eggs, soya beans, wholegrains including oatmeal, rye, brown rice.

Vitamin K

Required for: Bone building, essential for a blood-clotting compound known as prothrombin. (Given as an injection within first 15 minutes of birth to ensure adequate blood thickness as soon as baby is independent of the mother.) In puberty, can help reduce the severity of heavy menstrual bleeding.

Low levels may cause: No outward symptoms are likely to be seen.

Required daily doses:

Birth–6 months:	5 mcg
7 months–1 year:	10 mcg
1–3 years:	15 mcg
4–7 years:	20 mcg
8 years–puberty:	30 mcg rising to 55mcg in girls and 65 mcg in boys
Best food sources:	Bio yoghurt, egg yolks, fish oils, dairy produce and green leafy vegetables.

WATER SOLUBLE VITAMINS

Measured in milligrams (mg)

Vitamin B1

Required for: Energy production, carbohydrate digestion, cardiovascular and heart function, the nervous system and mental clarity and function.

Low levels may cause: Lethargy, lack of concentration, irritability, depression in older children.

Required daily doses:

Birth–6 months:	0.1 mg rising to 0.4 mg
6 months–1 year:	0.5 mg
1–3 years:	0.7 mg
4–7 years:	0.9 mg
8 years–puberty:	1.0 mg rising to 1.1 mg in girls and 1.3 mg in boys.
Best food sources:	Wholegrains, including oats, rye, millet and quinoa, legumes, dried yeast, liver and pork.

Vitamin B2

Required for: Digestion and metabolism of carbohydrates, fats and proteins, production of energy, healthy skin, hair and nails, development of sex organs, stress management.

Low levels may cause: Dry skin, cracked corners of mouth, red eyes.

Required daily dose:

Birth–6 months:	0.4 mg
6 months–1 year:	0.5 mg
1–3 years:	0.8 mg
4–7 years:	1.1 mg
8 years–puberty:	1.2 mg rising to 1.3 for girls and 1.5 mg for boys
Best food sources:	Bio yoghurt, fish, liver, milk, cottage cheese, green leafy vegetables.

Vitamin B3

Required for: Production of sex hormones and hormones relating to digestion of food and conversion into glucose (blood sugar management, insulin release, and thyroid hormones regulating metabolism). Mood regulation, brain function and nervous system.

Low levels may cause: Irritability, fatigue, lack of motivation and concentration, insomnia and blood sugar imbalances.

Required doses:

Birth–6 months:	5 mg
6 months–1 year:	6 mg
1–3 years:	9 mg
4–7 years:	12 mg
8 years–puberty:	13 mg rising to 15 mg for girls and 17 mg for boys

Vitamin B5

Required for: Most important for the support of the adrenal glands, which regulate the stress responses in the body. Needed for conversion of fats and carbohydrates into glucose for energy, and vital for the immune and nervous systems. Particularly important for the health of the ear, nose and throat passageways.

Low levels may cause: Frequent infections, irritability, poor blood sugar management and mood fluctuations.

Required daily doses:

Birth–6 months:	2 mg
6 months–1 year:	3 mg
1–3 years:	3 mg
4–7 years:	4 mg
8 years–puberty:	5–7 mg
Best food sources:	Wholegrains including rye, wheat, barley and millet. Nuts, chicken, egg yolks, liver, green vegetables.

Vitamin B6

Required for:	Immune, brain and nervous systems, digestion of proteins, all growth and repair in the body (works synergistically with zinc).
Low levels may cause:	Depression, mood swings, PMT in girls, anaemia, skin complaints.

Required daily doses:

Birth–6 months:	0.5 mg
6 months–1 year:	0.6mg
1–3 years:	1 mg
4–7 years:	1.1 mg
8 years–puberty:	1.4 mg–1.7 mg
Best food sources:	Chicken and other poultry, meats, liver, egg yolks, oily fish, leeks, kale, cabbage, dairy produce and wheatgerm.

Vitamin B12

Required for: (only visible after 6 months of insufficient intake)	Growth, digestion, brain and nervous function, especially concentration. Production of energy and manufacture of red blood cells.
Low levels may cause:	Anaemia, fatigue, ADHD and other attention disorders. Works with folic acid in cardiovascular system.

Required daily doses:

Birth–6 months:	0.3 mcg
6 months–1 year:	0.3–0.5 mcg
1–3 years:	0.7 mcg
4–7 years:	1.0 mcg
8 years–puberty:	1.4 mcg rising to 2.0 mcg
Best food sources:	red meat (liver, beef, pork), fish and shellfish, eggs, dairy produce, spirulina.

Folic Acid (part of B complex)

Required for:	Building antibodies (immune system), protein and carbohydrate digestion, energy production, preventing anaemia, stopping neural tube defects in pregnancy.

Low levels may cause:	Poor appetite, anaemia, digestive complaints, fatigue, skin problems.

Required daily doses:

Birth–6 months:	25 mcg
6 months–1 year:	35 mcg
1–3 years:	50 mcg
4–7 years:	75 mcg
8 years–puberty:	100 mcg rising to 150 mcg
Best food sources:	Dark green leafy vegetables, egg yolks, apricots, carrots, pumpkins and squashes, avocados, cantaloupe melon, wholewheat and rye grains.

Biotin (one of the B complex)

Required for:	Healthy skin, hair and nails, digestion of fats and proteins and energy production.
Low levels may cause:	Skin complaints, thinning hair or slow hair growth, muscle cramps, chronic fatigue.

Required daily doses:

Birth–6 months:	10 mcg
6 months–1 year:	15 mcg
1–3 years:	20 mcg
4–7 years:	25 mcg
8 years–puberty:	30 mcg rising to 100 mcg
Best food sources:	Brown rice, nuts, brewers yeast, liver, egg yolks, fruits.

Vitamin C

Required for:	Immunity, heart and cardiovascular function, development of sex hormones, stress management, skin tissue health (including gums and digestive tract as well as outer skin), wound healing.
Low levels may cause:	Poor wound healing, dry skin and other skin complaints, frequent infections and viruses, bleeding gums.
Required daily doses	Remember that the body cannot store vitamin C, so it is vital to ensure a regular supply through foods.
Birth–6 months:	30 mg
6 months–1 year:	35 mg
1–3 years:	40 mg
4–7 years:	45 mg
8 years–puberty:	45 mg rising to 60 mg (or more if your adolescent starts smoking. It is estimated that every cigarette wipes out 15 mg of usable vitamin C in the body!).

| **Best food sources:** | Berries, citrus fruits, kiwis, potatoes, squash and pumpkin, green leafy vegetables, sweet peppers, cabbage, broccoli, cauliflower, spinach. |

MINERALS

Calcium

| **Required for:** | Building healthy bones and teeth, cardiovascular and heart function, muscle contraction, nervous system. Works with iron. |
| **Low levels may cause:** | Muscle cramps, constipation, irritability and insomnia. |

Required daily doses:

Birth–6 months:	400 mg
6 months–1 year:	600 mg
1–3 years:	800 mg
4–7 years:	800 mg
8 years–puberty:	800 mg rising to 1000mg
Best food sources:	Green leafy vegetables, almonds, salmon, soya products.

Iron

| **Required for:** | Growth and development, red blood cell production, carrying oxygen to the brain and other organs. Works with calcium and B complex vitamins. |
| **Low levels may cause:** | Fatigue, anaemia, insomnia, sensitivity to the cold. |

Required daily doses:

Birth–6 months:	6 mg
6 months–1 year:	10 mg
1–3 years:	10 mg
4–7 years:	10 mg
8 years–puberty:	Rising to 15 mg in girls (more when menstruating), 13 mg in boys.
Best food sources:	Liver, peaches, apricots, raisins, figs and dates, egg yolks, red meat, nuts, bananas, avocados, parsley, watercress, spinach, kale, broccoli.

Magnesium

| **Required for:** | Regulates stress management, energy production, carbohydrate digestion, muscle, heart and nervous system function, and brain and mental functions. Works with calcium in bone formation and heart function, relief of menstrual cramps in adolescent girls. |

| **Deficiency symptoms:** | Hyperactivity and restlessness, twitchy leg syndrome, muscle cramps, depression and irritability. |

Low levels may cause:

Birth–6 months:	40 mg
6 months–1 year:	60 mg
1–3 years:	80 mg
4–7 years:	120 mg
8 years–puberty:	170 mg rising to 180 mg for girls.
Best food sources:	All green vegetables, citrus fruits, sweetcorn, almonds, mushrooms, nuts and seeds, figs, raisins, carrots, tomatoes, onions and garlic.

Selenium

| **Required for:** | Immune system, viral protection, skin health. Works with vitamin E. |
| **Low levels may cause:** | Dry skin, dandruff, skin problems, poor wound healing, frequent colds and infections. |

Required daily doses:

Birth–6 months:	10 mcg
6 months–1 year:	12 mcg
1–3 years:	20 mcg
4–7 years:	25 mcg
8 years–puberty:	30–45 mcg
Best food sources:	Shellfish, sesame seeds, wheatgerm and bran, tomatoes, broccoli and brazil nuts.

Zinc

| **Required for:** | Immune system, protein digestion and energy production, sexual organ and hormone development, brain function, nervous system and mood regulation, wound healing. |
| **Low levels may cause:** | Pale skin, poor wound healing, stunted growth, frequent infections, white flecks on fingernails, loss of taste or smell, rash around mouth and/or anus. |

Required daily dose:

Birth–12 months:	5 mg
1–3 years:	10 mg
4–7 years:	10 mg
8 years–puberty:	12 mg for girls and 15 mg for boys.
Best food sources:	Red meats, fish and shellfish, poultry, wholegrains, nuts and seeds, egg yolks, dairy produce, oats, rye, buckwheat, brown rice.

Resources

Nutritional supplements

Biocare
Lakeside, 180 Lifford Lane
King's Norton
Birmingham B30 3NU
Tel. 0121 433 3727
www.biocare.co.uk
An excellent range of vitamins and
minerals for breastfeeding mothers, babies
and children, multi-vitamins and mineral
powders, oils and fish oils, liquid vitamins
and mineral drops; no additives or artificial
ingredients.

Enzyme Process
4 Broadgate House, Westlode Street
Spalding PE11 2AF
Tel. 01775 761927
Email: enzymepro@compuserve.com
www.enzymepro.co.uk
Suppliers of Muc Liquescence and VIR
homeopathic drops.

Health Plus Ltd
Dolphin House, 30 Lushington Road
Eastbourne
East Sussex BN21 4LL
Tel. 01323 737374
www.healthplus.co.uk
Health Plus Pregnancy Pack: supplements
designed for before, during and after
pregnancy; also available from good
health-food stores.

Higher Nature Plc
The Nutrition Centre,
Burwash Common
East Sussex TN19 7LX
Tel. 0870 066 0808
www.highernature.co.uk
Mail order for children's chewable
multi-vitamins, essential balance oil and
flaxseed oil.

The Nutri Centre
7 Park Crescent
London W1N 3HE
Tel. 020 7436 5122
Email: enq@nutricentre.com
www.nutricentre.com

Quest Vitamins
8 Venture Way, Aston Science Park
Birmingham B7 4AP
Tel. 0121 359 0056
www.questvitamins.co.uk

Specialized formula milks

Organico
60–62 King's Road
Reading RG1 3AA
Tel. 0118 951 0518
Email: info@organico.co.uk
www.organico.co.uk
Babynat organic milk.

Vitacare Ltd
Unit One
7 Chalcot Road
London NW1 8LH
Tel. 0800 328 5826
'Nanny': nanny-goat milk, infant nutrition

Organic food suppliers

Stamp Collection
Buxton Food Limited
12 Harley Street
London W1G 9PG
Tel. 020 7637 5505
www.buxtonfoods.com
Mail-order gluten-free and dairy-free
products; gluten-free flours and breads also
available at most supermarkets.

Swaddles Green Farm
Hare Lane
Buckland St Mary
Chard
Somerset TA20 3JR
Tel. 01460 234387
www.swaddles.co.uk
Nationwide mail-order organic meat, game
and groceries, as well as pre-prepared
meals and children's food.

Village Bakery
Melmerby
Penrith
Cumbria CA10 1HE
Tel. 01768 881515
www.village-bakery.com

Other food and health organizations

The Anaphylaxis Campaign
PO Box 275
Farnborough
Hampshire GU14 6SX
Tel. 01252 542029
www.anaphylaxis.org.uk

The Asthma Society
Providence House, Providence Place
London N1 0NP
Tel. 020 7226 2260
www.asthma.org.uk

Biolab Ltd
The Stone House , 9 Weymouth Street
London W1W 6DB
Tel. 0207 636 5959
www.biolab.co.uk

British Allergy Foundation
Deepdene House
30 Bellegrove Road, Welling
Kent DA16 3PY
Tel. 0208 303 8525
Helpline: 0208 303 8583
www.allergyuk.org

British Association for Nutritional Therapies
(BANT)
27 Old Gloucester Street
London WC1N 3XX
Tel. 0870 606 1284
www.bant.org.uk

British Dietetic Association
5th Floor, Charles House
148–149 Great Charles Street
Queensway
Birmingham B3 3HT
Tel. 0121 200 8080
Email: info@bda.uk.com
www.bda.uk.com

British Nutrition Foundation
High Holborn House
52–4 High Holborn
London WC1V 6RQ
Tel. 020 7404 6504
www.nutrition.org.uk

British Society for Allergy and
Environmental and Nutritional Medicine
(BSAENM)
PO Box 28, Totton
Southampton SO40 2ZA
Tel. 0238 081 2124
Has a list of doctors who practise
nutritional and environmental medicine.

Children's Society
Edward Rudolf House
69–85 Margery Street
London WC1 XOJL
Tel. 020 7841 4400
www.childrenssociety.org.uk
Provides information about dealing with
underweight babies.

Coeliac Society
PO Box 220, High Wycombe
Buckinghamshire HP11 2HY
Tel. 01494 437 278
www.coeliac.co.uk

Department for Environment, Food and
Rural Affairs (DEFRA)
9 Millbank
c/o 17 Smith Square
London SW1P 3JR
Tel. 08459 33 55 77
Email: helpline@defra.gsi.gov.uk
www.defra.gov.uk
Central contact point for government
information on food issues.

Eating Disorders Association
1st Floor
Wensum House
103 Prince of Wales Road
Norwich NR1 1DW
Tel. 0845 634 1414
Youth helpline: 0845 634 7650
www.edauk.com

Food Commission
94 White Lion Street
London N1 9PF
Tel. 0207 837 2250
www.foodcomm.org.uk

Food Standards Agency
Aviation House, 125 Kingsway
London WC2B 6NH
Tel. 020 7276 8000
Email: helpline@foodstandards.gsi.gov.uk
www.food.gov.uk

Foresight
28 The Paddocks, Godalming
Surrey GU7 1XD
Tel. 01483 427839
www.foresight-preconception.org.uk
Natural pre-conceptual care; also provides
information on additives in food.

The Healthy House
The Old Co-op, Lower Street
Ruscombe, Stroud
Gloucestershire GL6 6BU
Tel. 01453 752 216
www.healthy-house.co.uk
Suppliers of allergy-free clothing, bedding
and other household items.

Hyperactive Children's Support Group
71 Whyke Lane, Chichester
West Sussex PO19 2LD
Tel. 01903 725182

Institute for Optimum Nutrition (ION)
13 Blades Court, Deodar Road
Putney, London SW15 2NU
Tel. 020 8877 9993
www.ion.ac.uk
A registered charitable trust for the study,
research and practice of nutrition.

La Leche League (LLL[GB])
PO Box 29, West Bridgford
Nottingham NG2 7NP
Tel. 020 7242 1278
www.laleche.org.uk
Offers breastfeeding support and
information.

National Childbirth Trust
Alexandra House, Oldham Terrace
London W3 6NH
Tel. 0870 444 8707
www.nctpregnancyandbabycare.com

National Eczema Society
NES, Hill House
Highgate Hill
London N19 5NA
Tel. 0870 241 3604
www.eczema.org

Parentline Plus
520 Highgate Studios,
57–79 Highgate Rd
Kentish Town
London NW5 1TL
Tel. 0808 800 2222
www.parentlineplus.org.uk

Society of Homeopaths
4A Artizan Road
Northampton NN1 4HU
Tel. 01604 621400
www.homeopathy-soh.org

Soil Association
Bristol House
40–56 Victoria Street
Bristol BS1 6BY
Tel. 0117 914 2400
www.soilassociation.org
The UK's leading campaigning and
certification body for organic food
and farming; the directory *Where to
buy Organic Food* contains details of
farm shops, box-delivery schemes and
local retailers.

Vegan Society
Donald Watson House
7 Battle Road
St Leonards on Sea
East Sussex TN37 7AA
Tel. 01424 427393
www.vegansociety.com

Vegetarian Society
Parkdale
Dunham Road
Altrincham
Cheshire WA14 4QG
Tel. 0161 925 2000
www.vegsoc.org

Index